DAVID M. FLANAGAN

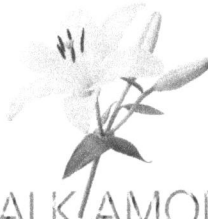

TO WALK AMONG
GRAVE
STONES

Personal Insights into Sobriety and the Search for a More Meaningful Life.

© *2019 David M. Flanagan*
Sacramento, California
First Edition

S-Club Publishing
1631 Alhambra Blvd – Suite 120
Sacramento, California 95816

ISBN: 978-0-578-48905-6

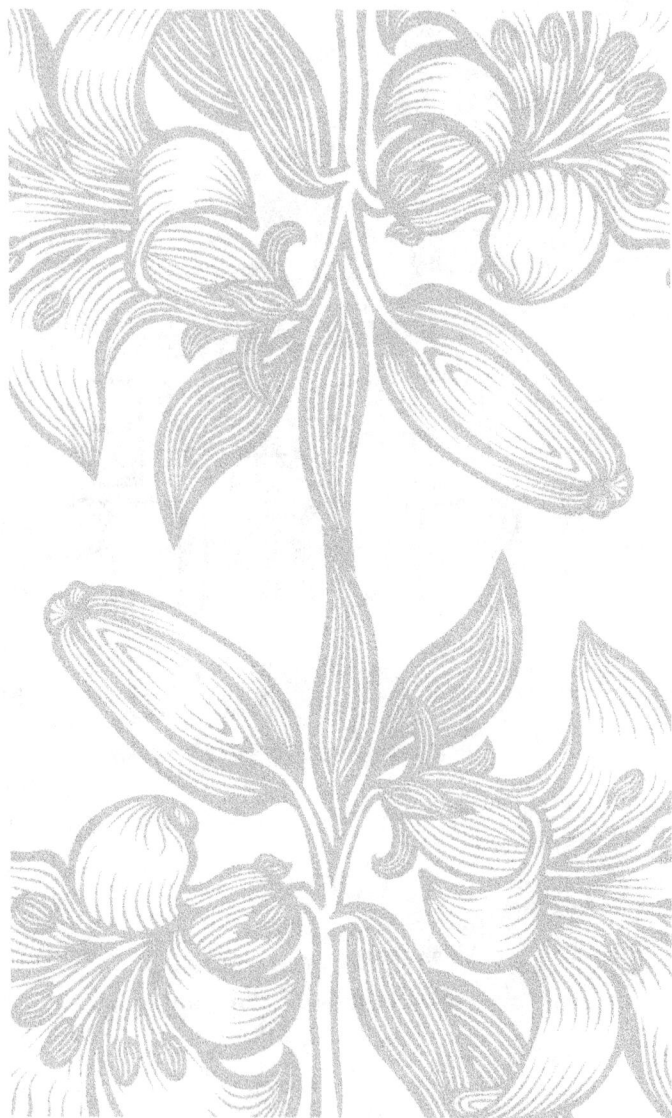

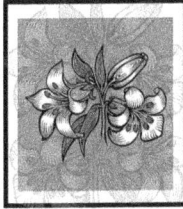

WHAT JUST HAPPENED?

———

SEPTEMBER 19, 2016

———

I woke up on the cold, cement floor of a dirty, downtown jail cell. My eyes welded shut, swollen and red, evidently, I had been there, virtually comatose the entire night. I didn't remember a single thing.

Nothing.

I had no idea of how I got there, and worse, what I did to deserve it. I take that back, I had a very good idea of why I was there, but as to the specific details, my mind and my recollection were a completely blank canvas. The only comfort, strangely enough, was that I had been here before. The same exact cement floor, actually. Twice. And with that understanding, realized, I was in big trouble…

———

They say God never gives us more than we can handle at one time...

Fortunately, He also never tells us in advance what He has in store for us, either, or about that huge bus barreling down the road directly at us.

If I had any indication, even a glimpse of what was to unfold in 2017, the unbelievable crap-storm and the life-altering, traumatic events...
I would have seriously considered jumping out of an airplane with no parachute on my back.

TABLE OF CONTENTS

TABLE OF CONTENTS

INTRODUCTION

If you've picked up this book, chances are you've had a few issues in your life surrounding alcohol, or the abuse of it, more specifically. I once had a counselor tell me, *"If alcohol has caused problems in your life… you have a problem with alcohol."*

I like this way of looking at the issue, because so many people, myself included for most of my adult life, refuse to acknowledge they even have a drinking problem. It sounds so gross. So sick. I sure as hell didn't want to be associated with those scum, low-life alcoholics who ruin their lives and everybody's around them. I was better than that. Far better. (In my own mind, anyway.)

So, soft-selling the issue, coming to the conclusion and admission that I had a "problem" with alcohol, made it somehow more palatable, regardless of the degree of that problem.

As it turns out, with booze, I had a pretty severe and growing problem. And that's what this book is about; how I have learned to recognize it, accept it, and deal with it. Call me an alcoholic or just a guy who never learned how to drink responsibly, but now, from a position of far greater clarity, I can see the road I have traveled and that perhaps, in some small way, I can shine a light on it for you as well.

In the coming chapters I will take you through the nightmare that unfolded for me over the course of 2017. I will delve into my past, for reference, but for the most part, my focus is on this one single, extremely painful year and how I was able to get through it, along with a staggering host of other new problems that surfaced along the way, and did so, for the first time in my life, without turning to a vodka tonic for friendly advice and emotional support.

In addition, scattered in between my own adventure, I will explore some rather unusual true stories of other people, some I know, some I knew, and some whom I never even met, having traveled equally difficult paths in their lives long before I was born.

In the end, I would like to believe my journey, yesterday and today, will provide you a glimpse of hope that perhaps you, too, might be able to gain a new and clearer perspective on your life and the possibility that you can actually face it, no matter how difficult, painful, or impossible that might seem, and do so…without your best friend, booze.

Trust me, I know how close one can become with a good stiff drink. Or five. A drink solves so many problems, even with the first sip. I loved so many things about drinking. The relaxation. The friends. The laughter. Unfortunately, it started adding far more problems than it ever solved, and as they started stacking up, overtaking my life, I knew someday I would have to quit. That day was forced upon me, so to speak, or at least called my name so loudly, that for once I actually listened.

So, if you can keep an open mind and truly listen to the story behind my story…I think you will find that, even as different as it is, it is also the same as yours. If alcohol is not your problem, I still feel strongly that the ways in which I am learning to deal with all the hurdles and potholes life seems to place in my path, will also work to see life not as an unfair game in which you always seem to lose, rather, a journey, filled with both pain and pleasure, and one that we can learn to embrace and cherish, no matter what comes our way.

For those struggling with alcohol, for those in jail because of it, for those who have destroyed their families and lost people they love, for those who have taken the lives of others as a result of a single drunken binge, and for those who are still perfectly happy with their drinking and cannot see how it has adversely affected them in any way, yet... I promise not to preach at you.

I am no one to offer answers to your life. I don't know anything about anything. I just have traveled a long and twisting road and think that maybe, some of the things I've seen along the way, might just be of interest to you. Maybe even helpful.

That is my hope.

So, opinionated and sarcastic as I am, please take these words as my story, not as a message of doom and gloom, or that I am fixed and now consider myself better than you in any way, shape or form. In reality, I know we are exactly the same. Different stories. Different roads. But both people. Both struggling to figure this weird world out. Both wanting happiness.

———

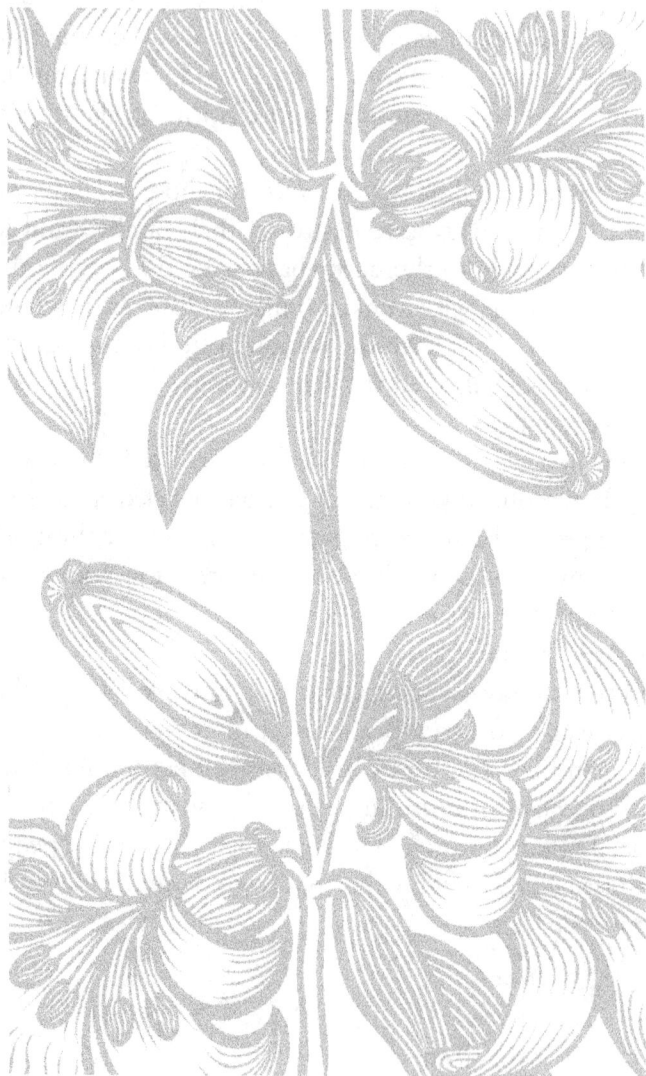

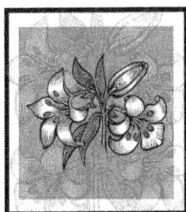

HOLY CRAP, I'M IN BIG TROUBLE NOW

———

SEPTEMBER 20, 2016

———

A jail is a horrible place. It stinks. Combine a collection of some of the absolute worst human odors in one tiny cement box, let it bake for days on end, and you will come close to recreating the daily ambiance of a jail cell. It's likely one of the most depressing, humiliating environments in which you might find yourself. And, where I found myself.

Surrounded by an unruly, extremely hungover group of men in my same situation, I managed to wake myself and sit up against the cold, gray wall. A small aluminum toilet was overflowing onto the floor and down a moldy drain, stuffed with toilet paper and excrement. The wall behind it was permanently stained, dripping with urine. Men laughed at unheard jokes trying to lighten their mood. Others still slept. Some, just sat quietly, rubbing their heads, wallowing in thick despair. I knew their thoughts.

But still, hard as I tried, there was no memories of the night before, absolutely zero. All I could recall was a late afternoon business meeting, a client, laughing and carrying on, enjoying each other's company, one cocktail, two cocktails, three. Then, maybe a few more. And after that, it was anyone's guess. I had experienced increasing black-outs over the previous years, but this was by far, the worst.

We were roused from our stupor and guided single file, out into a processing room. It was so damn bright. There were lights, neon and menacing, everywhere. They lined us all up, facing the wall and called us each by name, one after the other. I was handed my belongings, cell phone, wallet, and the contents of my pockets taken and bagged the previous night, handed a pile of legal paperwork, court documents, and other important information about what I inevitably faced next, then not-so-politely kicked out the door onto the street.

Downtown. Dark still. Cold. The city slowly coming to life. Maybe four or five in the morning. I still have no idea. At least I was out of the rat hole. My cell phone was dead, and my wife, Karin, had no idea either, where I was or what had happened and likely, feared the worst. Fortunately, my business office was only a few blocks away, so making the brisk excursion on foot, medicinal in a way, helping to wake up my clouded brain, I found relatively quick and familiar refuge to hunker down and sleep in safe privacy. Still, the memories of the night before were nonexistent. Blank. Empty. The fear began to creep in. What had I done? What had happened? What was going to happen?

I made my way to my office and let myself in, climbing the stairs, and went directly to the phone, calling Karin, to apologize and let her know I was at least alive. She said very little in return, in fact, if memory serves me now, I think she mumbled, "OK" and hung up. Falling back onto a leather couch, the pain eased ever-so-slightly, and I passed out once again.

Around 8:30 the office began to stir as staff members reported for their daily responsibilities and normal job routines. It was just another day for them. I'm not sure what they thought, but for those early morning folks, they certainly noticed that the boss was fully dressed, in the same rumpled clothes he had on the day before, crashed on the couch in his office. Not a pretty picture to say the least. I woke up, suddenly very aware that I could not be seen in this way, not now, not like this, and made a rather quick exit, not greeting anyone, making eye contact, or saying a thing.

I bolted for the door.

Out on the street once again, the sun had risen now and was far brighter than before, shocking my puffy eyes. Damn, what had I done this time? I didn't know which direction to head. I stood there, rubbing my head, turning in a circle, confused. I must have appeared to the normal working crowd now filling the streets as one of the many homeless people who color the downtown sidewalks. Candidly, the only difference was that I had a home to go home to.

I had absolutely no idea where my car was, so I simply started walking in the direction of home. My stomach, despite a rather monstrous hangover, was growling in hunger, and the sudden thought of a hot breakfast seemed to call my name.

I made my way on foot, somehow, to a local restaurant, sat out on the balcony and ordered eggs, bacon, a mound of fried potatoes and buttered toast. The hot coffee went down easily. It was like a good dose of overdue medicine, even if it did nothing to help my incredible hangover. The only thing that made it better, was the double Bloody Mary I drank to wash it all down. Along with the second. My self-abuse was not finished yet, evidently, and so I used this (last) opportunity to completely vanquish the growing pain in my mind and that chastising, echoing threat; the dark, menacing, ever-increasing voice of terror.

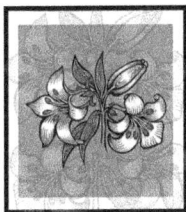

UM, A LITTLE HELP, HERE?

SEPTEMBER 5, 2016

"God... " I whispered in torment, *"I need help."* Backing up just a hair, before this whole shit storm came crashing down on my head, those were my exact words I spoke, out loud, and I meant them like I'd never meant anything before. Whether you believe in God, the Universe, Zeus, whatever... call it what you will, but roughly two weeks prior to getting tossed in jail for driving under the influence, I had actually reached out for help.

Evidently, despite common opinions to the contrary, God sometimes listens.

I'm not sure how, but I remember clearly, sitting on my living room couch with one of those more ruthless kind of hangovers; the ones where you wished you'd drank at least one glass of water before bed, but didn't, and would defiantly offer your middle finger to the world, heading directly back to bed. Only this time, I couldn't. Another important meeting or some pressing deadline, I had to go to work, so, manned-up, groaning like a water buffalo stuck in the mud, and made my best effort to get dressed.

Sitting there, though, struggling just to tie my shoes, I was wracked with a severe pounding headache and this disgusting overall queasiness surging throughout my entire body resembling, I imagine, how many people feel after endless days tossed about on a stormy sea.

I just couldn't handle it anymore. Of course, this wasn't the first time I'd pressed on through a hangover. Hardly. I'd been right here, moaning in pain, sitting on the same damn couch, tying my shoes before. I had done this so many countless times. When was it going to stop? Oh, I had tried to change, trust me. I had tried to quit drinking, many times. A few of which, I had even shown signs of success, stopping for a few weeks, but always, always coming back. My intentions were pretty good. My resolve sucked.

As I had been told in my youth, the road to hell is paved with good intentions.

And so, in a moment of desperation, I just blurted out the words. "God, I need help…" As soon as they left my lips, however, I burst into nervous laughter. (Strange, I know) But, I immediately held up my finger and, out loud, followed my little heartfelt prayer with an escape clause. "Wait! Wait… I take that back," I said. "I know Your kind of help! And that is not what I'm talking about here." I sat there for a few minutes longer, silently, thinking about what had just taken place. I think I just prayed…like a real prayer. And worse still, I think I could actually hear His answer, too.

"So…do you want help, or do you not want help?"

I smiled to myself, realizing that if I truly believed in a God who loved me, and I was asking for His help, then maybe, just maybe, I should trust Him to help me in whatever way he saw fit. "Not my will but thine be done" and all that King James biblical stuff. After all, up to this point, I certainly hadn't been able to help myself.

Over the years, my drinking grew steadily worse, daily, often ending in severe drunkenness by the time I made it home. Client meetings with cocktails, staff celebrations at the office for no particular reason, catching up with old friends, or just a quick martini or three all by myself, I often started drinking by noon.

"Ok, Ok… Yes, I need help," I continued. "Go ahead. Do whatever it is you do…"

From there, I slowly finished tying my shoes and clambered off to one more painful day at the office, forgetting all about my little conversation with my Maker. Evidently, He didn't forget though. As it turns out, it seems He took my little outburst quite seriously.

Interestingly, I've prayed many, many times over the years, always falling on deaf ears it seemed. Thousands of unanswered prayers. But for some reason, God only knows (pun intended), He took special note of this short little cry for help, proceeded to grab a large baseball bat from some dusty closet up in Heaven, and beat the living snot out of me.

———————————

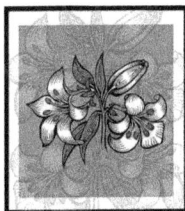

The Living Nightmare of
MAREN CONRAD

"You're a total idiot", **Maren's sister chided.** *"Guys like this are what every girl dreams about. You've got one, literally begging you to go out with him, and you said... no?"*

It was true, according to Maren, all signs pointed to Dennis Conrad, a very alluring man she had recently met, potentially being the man of her dreams. But, seriously, it was all a little too good to be true. She was, after all, just a simple bartender. He was a successful VP at Morgan Stanley. She was a starving artist. He was a wealthy financier. Salt and pepper, the two did not appear to fit. "Charming, rich, good looking, and so sweet," she recalls, "of all the people on earth, why would he be even remotely interested in me?" And yet, he was…

One simple dinner date rolled rather rapidly into the sound of wedding bells and a classic fairytale romance that exploded like apple blossoms in Spring. A storybook ceremony at the Alhambra Palace in Granada, Andalusia, Spain was followed by a feast set for kings in a classic Flamenco cave. Add an exquisite Italian honeymoon and Maren's world suddenly became a bit unbelievable. An unexpected gift. A grateful miracle. Then, when it couldn't possibly get any better, a touch of frosting on her cake, Hunter, an angelic baby boy entered the picture, creating a whole new level of utter sublime bliss.

How things can change with a few ticks of the clock.

The three of them became inseparable. "Every day at 5:30, baby Hunter and I would sit on the front porch of our beautiful home", Maren recalls, a tear in her eye, "waiting for Daddy to come home." But this life, as incredible as it had become, was not to last. Suddenly, just as quickly as it began, the dream was over.

Running late for their daily homecoming, Maren noticed the garage door was wide open. Stranger still, Dennis' car was not in the driveway either. Numerous warning signs, as loud as they were, became clouded and ignored, including the bright red drops of blood lining the kitchen floor.

Turning the corner into the living room, Maren was met with the unimaginable sight of her husband, lying face down, in a massive pool of his own blood. Hunter still strapped in the car outside, she went for the phone to dial 911, but it was missing. Only then did she begin to notice the entire house had been ransacked. Broken, smashed, turned upside down, some madman had broken into her home and destroyed her world. Dennis had paid the price.

Finding another phone, she managed to call 911, returning immediately to her husband, administering mouth-to-mouth; a natural instinct, but futile effort. Dennis was gone. The police found Maren in shock, her face and clothes covered in blood.

The fear, anguish, and utter humiliation that followed were, as Maren recalls, surreal.

"They took hundreds of pictures of me," she says. "I can understand now, just doing their job, they thought I might have done it."

Luckily, having stolen their car as well, authorities were able to track the license plate and apprehend the killer in only a few hours — a seemingly random burglar, strung out on meth, with no understanding or concern for the beautiful family he had just destroyed.

The trial lasted for three long years. An unremorseful murderer, James Shanrock, appeared to be a total stranger seeking to support his habit. In a drug-induced frenzy, he actually emptied an entire bullet clip, took the time to reload, and just kept shooting at Dennis. In the back. Eleven times.

Maren was asked if she wanted to pursue the death sentence, an almost impossible question for a 25-year old. As much as she wished this man the same pain he had caused, she couldn't go as far. When he was given six life sentences without the possibility of parole, Maren simply closed her eyes and wept.

It was her husband's best friend (name withheld), who stood by her through the whole traumatic experience. As it turned out, however, Maren's nightmare was far from over, and his intentions were anything but honorable. In her state of emotional weakness, he wooed her, seduced her, conned her, and *convinced her to marry him. In doing so, she unwittingly handed over the keys of the kingdom to a veritable sociopath.*

Anything but a friend, he very calculatingly funded his own growing drug addiction, systematically selling all that she owned, draining savings accounts, trust fund accounts, life insurance settlements, even her son's college fund. Then, adding insult to injury, he racked up a line of credit on her house well over $600,000.

"He took everything I had left and then some," says Maren. The financial loss was nothing though, compared to the physical and verbal abuse that increasingly mounted, both to her and Hunter. "He would beat us both and I didn't know how to make it stop."

What kind of person could act this way? Who steps in on behalf of his murdered best friend, and destroys what is left? What does a man like this, upon looking in the mirror, say to himself? It is beyond comprehension.

"So, one day, I thought...I don't have to do this anymore," she says. "I walked out the door with Hunter and just left it all behind." With absolutely no idea how she would survive or put food on the table, Maren searched for odd jobs, teaching art at a few local schools, creating an occasional painting on commission, anything she could to manage. One of these pieces caught the attention of Elliot Fouts, owner of a Sacramento gallery, who asked if he might represent her. And just like that, once again, the clouds began to clear, the sun still there to shine down upon her.

Then, in a twist of fate nobody could have predicted, the impossible happened. One particular painting, The Persimmon Tree, was purchased by an admirer as a gift to his wife. "The persimmon," as Maren explains it, "is an intense, bright orange fruit, often covered in a layer of frost, brought forth in the freezing dead of winter." She had created this unique piece as a personal symbol of the incredible beauty often born from intense pain. Captured only by the image itself, the man who purchased the piece knew nothing of its deeper meaning nor had any prior knowledge of the painter who created it. His wife, on the other hand, now that was a different story altogether.

The Persimmon Tree, gracing the wall of their home, was seen by a visitor who took note, casually mentioning, "Oh, that's a Maren Conrad piece. What an incredible story she has..." Making no connection still, the visitor was pressed to reveal the underlying story of Maren's shocking past, the murder, the trial, and suddenly... it all hit home.

The woman to whom the painting had been given was none other than Sharon Chamisa, the public defense attorney who represented the cold-blooded killer of Maren's husband.

Sharon wrote Maren a long letter of abject apology, offering to return the painting. She only wanted to do the right thing. In her letter, she continued to explain that having to defend Shanrock was one of the most painful experiences of her entire life and resulted ultimately, in the choice to end her career as a trial lawyer. It had, in fact, completely devastated her.

Upon receiving the letter, Maren broke into tears and picked up the phone. Reopening the wound, yet somehow healing the pain, she gained a new and rather unexpected friend in the process. Shanrock, this soulless shell of a man, had shattered both of their lives. Some would consider this all a rather bizarre series of random coincidences. Others, like Maren, who don't believe in such coincidence...a very rare and precious miracle.

Since that time, Maren's life as a painter has catapulted forward. There has been no looking back. Her acclaim and status as a celebrated artist have skyrocketed. "My work is *hanging in galleries across the country now," she says in complete surprise. "In the Aerna Gallery, I'm actually hanging right next to Annie Leibovitz." And indeed, Maren's name has achieved rising notoriety. Many in her hometown of Sacramento have become increasingly familiar with her and the striking caliber of her work. Few know, however, in the dead of winter, the ice-covered road she traveled to get here.*

Married once again to an incredible man, Geoff Jernigan, whom Maren lovingly refers to as "Captain America," she holds tightly to the only thing she really values, hope. "Nobody can ever take that from me. Ever," she says, eyes filled light. "No matter what happens, Hunter and me…we will always come out on the other side. As for tomorrow, I have no goals," Maren offered, rather matter-of-factly. "Goals are things people put in place in an effort to live tomorrow. I'm perfectly happy right where I am, simply living today."

Then, as the conversation drew to an end, Maren offered one more small insight that seemed to sum up her entire story.

"My life is a painting," she said. "I love the actual process of painting itself, not the end product. If I have to worry about how a painting will end up, how it will turn out, that's way too scary. I would never even start. I'm not attached to outcomes anymore." She paused briefly, then finished with,

"I just paint.
Then I paint some more."

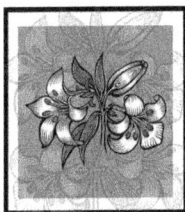

TIME TO COME CLEAN

———

SEPTEMBER 28, 2016

———

It may sound shallow, but one of the biggest hurdles I faced, was psychological. I was horribly embarrassed about the whole fiasco. After all, I was an established, respectable businessman with clients and influential community associates. I served on charity boards. I was a father, a husband, a brother and a son. All these people, I couldn't let them know the truth about me…that I was, in the shadows, an alcoholic and a criminal.

The utter humiliation ate away at me. Again, call it what you will, it was very real to me. It took me a while, but the best medicine I could find to alleviate the pain, was simply coming clean. Step out of the shadows and confess my sins.

My wife, Karin, of course, already knew. My brother, John, was next in line, and strangely, one of the most difficult people to talk to about it. As my older brother and best friend, I craved his acceptance, respect and admiration. I had tried to hide my drinking problem from him over the years and, as a result, it only served to create a growing division, a wall, between us. A candid conversation, the truth, then broke it all down. Talking to him about it was like a breath of fresh air.

We sat together in my backyard for hours just talking about our childhood, our unique friendship through the years, the struggles we both faced as adults, and our desire to challenge the world together. It was one of the best conversations I can ever remember having. And it changed me. It cleansed me, just a little, and instilled no small amount of strength to move through the fire that was waiting for me still, just ahead.

Using this experience as a source of inspiration and new strength, I slowly began to open the door and tell others, those to whom I was close, what had happened and who I really was. My mother and other siblings. My business partner, Matt. Close friends. Long-time business associates. The more I stepped forward with the brutal truth, the freer I felt and the stronger I became in my resolve not to drink anymore as well as the seemingly insurmountable difficulties and trials I was now facing.

Another repeated hurdle was that of clients. In the industry of advertising and marketing, my chosen professional field, life more often than not revolves around the gathering for cocktails. Over and over, I now had to reject invitations to get together after hours over a beer or a drink. Naturally, accustomed to me being the one to initiate such meetings, many were more than curious.

Without revealing the entire ugly story, I managed to begin to tell the simple truth, that I had stopped drinking, as a way to redirect meetings. I began to suggest early morning cups of coffee instead. If that sounds a bit boring, I would have agreed prior to my experience. While I love a good cup of coffee as much as the next guy, nothing could beat a cold martini. But strangely enough, turning to coffee conversations instead, especially the first thing in the day, set a whole new outlook. More got accomplished. My days became far more productive. I didn't really lose any respect, rather gained a little, perhaps.

I can't say it's been a perfect turnaround. There are still difficult situations which I admit, I try to avoid rather than dealing with them head on. But they are growing farther and fewer in between. I'm getting better at orchestrating my daily life around things other than drinking. This alone, provided yet again a new source of strength to continue on my journey into sobriety. Something I had lost all hope of ever obtaining was now feasible and somehow within reach. Prior to this, the rather seductive voice of alcohol always there in my head, would reason with me and remind me, "There is no way you can be successful in your industry without booze..."

And I believed it.

It was a sense of hopeless acceptance. Everybody I knew drank. But it simply wasn't true. My life did not have to revolve around drinking. That voice in my head didn't care one bit about me, what happened to me, or how it might affect others, especially the ones I love most. It really only cared about getting one more drink and would tell me anything I needed to hear to make that happen.

Very sly, that voice. But once I began to step back and listen, to identify it for what it was, the stronger I became in telling it to shut the hell up. Seemingly so powerful when crouching in the dark, once exposed to the light, in this case simple recognition of the voice itself, the power it held over me weakened greatly.

But it was in the confession, the telling of my truth to others, that I began to grow and become increasingly stronger in my resolve. Transparency became a new and interesting life goal, freeing me in other, very unexpected ways. I had no idea how much I had been hiding from others and myself. In no small way, the more open I became about my drinking problem and new direction in life, the less stress I carried and the freer I became.

———

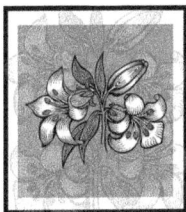

The Unplanned Detour of
KEVIN RAMOS

Kevin almost died the other day. One minute, relaxing in the comfort of his own living room, playing with a new puppy, allowing it to chomp on his fingers, and the next…fighting for his very life.

Change, real change, is not always something desirable, a goal to be pursued, or a prize to be won. Sometimes change is a dark, unfriendly shadow that just shows up on your doorstep and waltzes in to your home uninvited. It makes demands and gives you no choice. But your next move and how you end up dealing with those demands reveal what kind of person you are or, perhaps, shapes the kind of person you become.

Most of us don't like to think about the precarious nature of life, how much we take for granted, don't appreciate, and how quickly it can all be ripped from us. But Kevin Ramos, in his face-to-face visit with death, is no longer one of them. He tossed death right back out the front door and onto the lawn. Now he takes his life and every minute of the day as a gift. One to treasure. One to share.

"It came on very fast," Kevin recounted over a cup of coffee. Then he stopped, momentarily gathering his thoughts. "I don't really do this a lot, looking back," he said. "I prefer looking forward. But I guess it's good, now and then, to revisit all this. Sort of brings me back to reality."

This "reality" hit him like a rogue semi-truck barreling 100 miles per hour down the freeway in a fog bank. "Out of nowhere, these severe flu-like symptoms came on," he said. "104-degree temperature, intense aching, I went down…just out of the blue." With a slight sarcastic grin, he continued, "But I'm a man, right? I'm tough. So, I did what any man would do…I went to bed."

The next morning, however, it was clear that he had something far more than just the flu. His doctor, unfortunately, could not see him immediately. So he and wife, Kathleen, opted to make a mad dash to the local Urgent Care to be on the safe side. Smart decision, except that he was quickly diagnosed with the flu and sent directly back to square one. "Go home, drink plenty of water and get some rest. That'll be a hundred dollars, thank you very much. Next…"

Rest didn't help and Kevin's condition progressed steadily downhill. Straight off a sheer cliff is more like it. When the Tamiflu proved useless and he began to turn a lovely shade of purple, Kathleen dialed 911. His next visit was directly to the emergency room of Sutter Memorial. They were not so quick and cavalier in their diagnosis. Recognizing his symptoms for what they were, some sort of nasty infection, the ER crew took it a little more seriously and the game was on. The only questions were what kind of infection it was and...was it too late? By this time all of Kevin's internal systems had begun shutting down.

Then, boom, lights out. In the throes of severe sceptic shock, Kevin did not regain consciousness until four, long, terrifying weeks.

Four weeks. In that time, arm-wrestling non-stop with death, his family continually at his bedside, the medical team fought around the clock to save him. Two priests performed his Last Rights. And despite all of this, the chances of him surviving, well, let's just say, at an average of 5%...little if any. Hope was not a subject discussed lightly. Tears replaced make-up. Imminent funeral plans were likely offered. Brought on by something as innocent as a nip on the finger from his puppy, nobody is really sure, even healthy people just don't seem to survive these types of infections.

At a young 52 years old, Kevin steers the ship of the Buzz Oates Company, serving as their Chief Investment Officer. Not exactly a part-time summer job, it has been his domain for the last 22 years. With an incredible family of four children and a devoted wife of 26 years, you could say that Kevin was a man who had carved out a very successful life. He serves on the Board of Directors for Saint John's Program for Real Change, freely and abundantly giving his time, money and efforts to help others. By all accounts, he is a good man. Why then was this happening to him? What had he done to deserve such a painful tragedy? The answer is an equally painful...nothing. Nothing at all. This was simply a bad hand that life had dealt him. In every sense, fair or not, it appeared that it was his turn to go.

But Kevin, his family, friends, and the entire medical team vehemently disagreed. If it was his time to die, it certainly wasn't going to be without an all-out battle. As it turned out, it was a fight they never could have fathomed.

Infections lead to more infections. Problems created more problems. Guesswork and theory. Surgery and healing. Touch-and-go again and again. In an effort to save his brain and internal organs, he was administered a batch of complicated drugs that work to stabilize and centralize blood pressure, but unfortunately reduce blood flow to the extremities. Like a form of frostbite, hands, fingers, feet and toes grow ever colder. Then they die.

When the initial infection was finally defeated, the war had taken its toll on his body. Irreparable skin tissue was a concern. Brain damage was a constant threat. The battle was far from over. Waking up almost one month later, Kevin was given the news that he would lose two fingers, possibly even his hands and both legs, just below the knees. Non-negotiable. They had to go. How does a man receive news like this? How on Earth is someone supposed to recover from this?

"It wasn't really all that difficult to decide," says Kevin. "Having come so far, there was no choice but to continue. Others had certainly traveled this road. I thought...I can get there. Plus, by this point, I completely trusted the medical team...so, yeah, let's do it."

(I believe that's referred to as courage.)

As a hiker and a downhill ski enthusiast his whole life, the thought of losing his legs was not something he had ever considered. But suddenly, there it was. Deal with it, son.

So many of us, especially around the first of January each year, scribble down a short list of all the things we want to change about ourselves. Weight, career, relationships... they *could use some improvements. Some of the more noble among us make deeper, even spiritual decisions to improve their lot in life with heartfelt intention to finally shift gears, right the rudder, draw a line in the sand, and finally redirect our mismanaged lives. Sometimes successful, often not, that kind of change is something we decide we want, something we pursue, something we choose.*

Kevin, however, was not given a choice in the matter. Radical change came screaming into his living room like a demonic tornado and tossed him out of his chair onto the floor.

So again, the big question remains; How is a person supposed to deal with that? How do you survive, not just the physical part, but the horrific psychological aftermath? Something you never asked for and would never want in a million years. How could you ever regain all that you lost? And yet, somehow, that's exactly what Kevin decided to do. Regain as much of his life as he possibly could.

It became his motivation, his goal, his vindication. Two months after he had gone to bed with a fever, he returned home, in a wheelchair, missing fingers and two robotic aluminum poles where his legs once were.

But this is the part of the story where everything hinges, becoming nothing less than miraculous. This is actually where the story begins. As it turns out, Ottobock, a pioneering company that makes specialized prosthetic ski feet caught Kevin's attention. "I want that!" he mandated. "I want to ski again." And so it was that a rare infection and imminent death lost their arrogant grip on this strange man to the steep and seductive slopes of Heavenly Valley in South Lake Tahoe.

He drives his own car now, too. Equipped with sophisticated hand controls, you might even pass him on the freeway, never knowing that the cool-headed guy behind the wheel recently fought for his life and won.

"Airport security is a whole lot of fun too," he smirks. "I've often been asked if I'm a veteran and I have to admit, nothing quite that heroic. I wish I had more valor..."

True humility is a beautiful thing when you witness it.

He isn't shy about his space-age legs, either. Quite the opposite in fact. "I often wear shorts in public. The crowd tends to part like the Red Sea. It gives me more room," he laughs. "Things like this make people uncomfortable", he admits. "Everybody is curious, but nobody wants to stare. Except kids...they can't help themselves. I don't mind. It's a teachable moment. So, I always try to break the ice, crack a joke, just lighten the mood to take the pressure off."

Thinking about it momentarily, he smiled and offered, "Besides, if you can't have fun with something like this...you're missing out on a great opportunity."

Um, what?

What was that? Have fun with it? What kind of a weird life-philosophy is that? A perfectly healthy young man suddenly loses consciousness for a month, then wakes up, comes home in a wheel chair without multiple body parts, and his response... "Have fun with it or you're missing out on a great opportunity!" Incredible. I get depressed when my front lawn begins to turn brown. I don't know what religion he has, but I want it.

I pressed him further. Tell me more about your attitude. It's shockingly positive. Is this what got you through all this?

"Yeah, I guess," he offers, as though he'd never really given it much thought. "In hindsight, as traumatic as it all was, I see it now as more of a blessing than anything. It's made me better than I was."

At this point in our conversation, I stopped scribbling in my notepad, my mouth just hanging open. Maybe he really was a robot. I wanted to punch him.

"One big benefit that has come out of it all," he continued, "is my mind. I still have my mind. And it's calmer now. Mentally. I have this great life and tons and tons of support. In fact, its been a groundswell of people who love me. My boys…Nicholas, Frank, Carlin…my daughter, Kristen. And my wife, Kathleen…I wouldn't have made it without her. All my friends, co-workers…they all came together. I'm just so thankful. It's really cool."

Really cool. And thankful? You had your legs literally taken out from underneath you and your response…is you're thankful? I was not sure how to respond to such a statement. By this time in our conversation I felt like asking him if he would consider starting a spiritual commune or a religious movement of some sort. I'd follow him.

"I really want to run again," he confessed, as if he had still somehow failed. "And walk into the ocean like I used to. I really miss that. I want to get as much of my life back as I can, you know? Today can be pretty dark, but you never know what tomorrow might hold…"

We both sat in silence, allowing those powerful words to soak in. This had become one of the most inspirational conversations I have ever had. This very unusual man had faced the un-faceable and discovered some real answers to life. He was living them. And it showed.

"I do manage to hike a little still, although my endurance has declined, nine or ten miles at best," he confided, ashamed of himself. "The steep terrain is somewhat of a challenge."

Oh, please… now just stop!

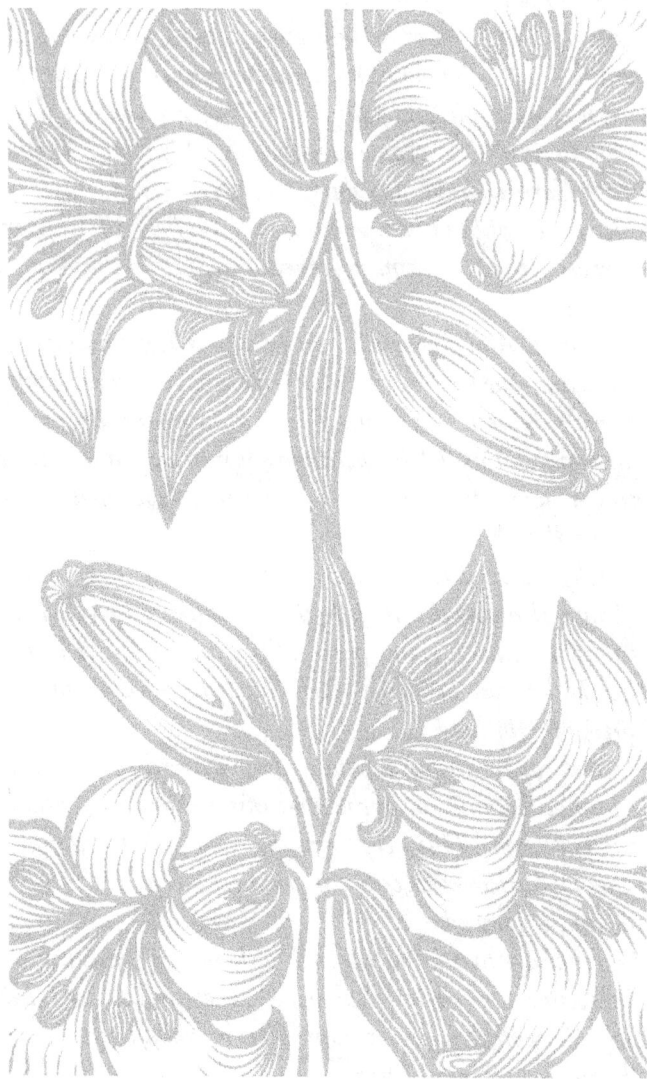

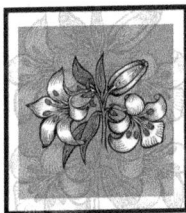

TRANSPORTATION AND GETTING AROUND

NOVEMBER 10, 2016

OK, life without a driver's license sucks. Now what? I seriously considered what many people choose, driving on a suspended license, but the truth is, I felt like I had caused enough trouble and pain already and was in more than enough hot water than I cared for. The thought of adding even more penalties or potentially even jail time to my sentence, was a rather convincing deterrent.

So, I bought a new bicycle.

Seen through one set of lenses, an old man riding a bicycle to work, in the wind and rain, is pretty sad. Depressing even. Trust me, I felt good and sorry for myself plenty of times. But then, seen from another perspective, another set of lenses, it's actually quite liberating in its simplicity. No gas. No parking. I lost fifteen pounds. After a while, a month or two, it became second nature to hop on the bike and go. It caused ongoing difficulties, getting to client meetings and more, but with a little creativity, I somehow was always able to work around it.

I remember one morning in particular, windy, cold and wet, I bundled up head-to-toe in a rain suit. It helped a little, but I still got wet. The rain coming down hard, it filled the brim of my hat and dripped right down in front of my face in a steady stream of water. I was pissed. I shouldn't be in this situation. I had fought my entire life, struggled to make something of myself, build businesses, feed my family, accomplish great things...and in the second half of my life, I was now forced to ride a freaking bike in the freezing rain just to get to work so I could pay my fines. Yeah, I was bent, depressed and really angry. At myself. There was nobody else to blame.

Yes, I often ridiculed the lame-ass justice department, whom I am still convinced cares nothing about helping people like me. All they are capable of doing is just hitting offenders with a big stick as hard as they can and removing as much money from their pockets as possible. There is no real concern. There is contempt not compassion. And despite the so-called "programs" mandated, there is zero intent to actually solve any issues or problems. It's a whole lot of bureaucratic bullshit red tape and that's not me feeling sorry for myself. That's actually, clear as a bell, just the facts. The current system, like so many (if not all) government, city, county systems, has no clue what they are doing and, in the end, doesn't really care. It's just a stupid job with a guaranteed pay raise, vacations, health benefits, and the promise of some sort of pension someday if they can last long enough. They stamp their documents and process paperwork in endless tidy little folders.

Uber. Now there's a company who knows how to solve a problem. There's someone who actually sat down and used their brain to create something that never existed before and actually eliminate a hurdle. They changed lives. They helped people. The current justice system could never, would never, be capable of creating a concept like *Uber.* To begin with, did I mention they just don't care?

I downloaded the app for *Lyft* but, for some reason, gravitated to using *Uber* on occasion. As the weather moved through summer, then into fall again, becoming colder, I began turning to the seemingly ever-present *Uber* drivers more and more.

At first, it was a bit awkward, climbing into somebody else's car, but it beats a bicycle in a rainstorm. I've never been a big taxi guy, small town attitude and all, so it was a bit of a personal hurdle, but I got over it. Within a very short amount of time, I grew to rely on the utter convenience. The drivers, as I mentioned, are everywhere. And I mean everywhere. I have never waited for a ride more than five minutes.

Uber has thought it through, top to bottom, and provides an incredible, seamless experience. It's amazing. If it had been created by the current justice system, it would have been introduced using a blind old man pushing a wheelbarrow around town. Sort of like a snail-paced, low-budget, rickshaw service. And the tax payers would have to foot the bill.

Here's an idea…one that the government could care less about. How about if we eliminate drunk driving 100% forever? How about we invent a technology that, starting tomorrow, would stop every single drunk driving accident and the thousands upon thousands of people's lives, families, children, parents, all those innocent souls who have perished because of someone's choice, or lack thereof, to drive under the influence? How about we just stop all that right now?

The technology is already available. But instead of using it to solve the problem, it has been instituted as a money-maker. The breath-a-lyzer. The ignition inter-lock. It effectively removes the threat of a car from running if it detects alcohol on the driver. Boom. Problem solved. Unfortunately, the current system mandates the use of these little devices long after the damage has already been done. After the crime has been committed. After someone has been caught, or worse, another killed.

Sorry, but that's a bit late.

Why doesn't every single car on the road have one of these devices in it? I'm sorry, I just don't understand. Seriously? The scope and size of the alcohol problem in our country? The devastating tragedies that have been seen? The over-packed jails? The tax payer dollars to support it all? And all of this, we could solve in about minute and a half?

The obvious answer, short-sighted and selfish as it is, would be the infringement on another's personal right to freedom. *"I don't drink, why should I have to have an alcohol system in my car?"* The answer is really quite simple, Bozo. Because drinking and driving is against the law. Just like driving without a seat belt is against the law. Or driving backwards on the freeway, blindfolded. These are not matters of personal freedom. They are laws.

Driving under the influence, however, is a law that when broken, is enforced too late and the result is often the death of another person. But it doesn't have to be that way. If it was enforced prior to driving, problem solved. No more dead people on the freeway at 2:00 in the morning. No more packed jail cells downtown. No more endless lines of people standing before a sleeping judge who himself is drunk. No more.

The technology is simple and sitting right smack in front of us. If you drink, you simply cannot start the engine. As a society, under the heavy-handed rule of a severely broken system, we simply have chosen to ignore it.

Now, I could go all dark, evil, and conspiracy-theory on you and try to convince you that the current system makes piles of cash off the drunk-driving problem, that they don't just lack the motivation to fix the problem, rather are financially motivated to perpetuate it…but I think I should probably just stick to the facts, even if my personal opinions are dead-on accurate. Who am I to suggest that our government, by and large, is an antiquated system of dead people who don't give a hoot about anybody? Like lifeless zombies, they chew on the bones of others, pocketing their fat, little paychecks each week. I wouldn't dare. Without showing how I really feel, it's safe to say that far too many state workers, not all, but many, do not do much of anything other than stamping pieces of paper with ink. I suppose there's a need for that.

If you're a state worker and my assessment absolutely does not apply to you, I either apologize or compliment you. You are rare, indeed. If it does apply to you, I hope you're good and mad. You should be ashamed of yourself.

———————————

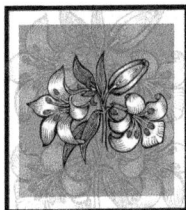

MY DAY IN COURT

———

DECEMBER 7, 2016

———

I hired an attorney. The same guy I hired last time I got a DUI. Jeff Rosenblum. Cool, Jewish guy who seems to drink rocket fuel for breakfast. Like a little bird, always moving, darting his head this way and that, Jeff has a sense of self-imposed urgency about him that causes you to feel like you better not waste even a half-second of his time. If you do, or if you begin to wander off the subject of his interest, he begins tapping his fingers and nervously looking at his watch.

Funny thing is, we had just bumped into each other several months prior at the funeral of a mutual friend's father. Sitting at the bar of all places. That was the one time I didn't see him tap his fingers.

It had been eight years since I'd seen Jeff. Eight years. In that time, the laws had changed and not in my favor. I had hoped, based on the laws in place during my prior DUI, that sufficient time had passed and that I would therefore only be facing what would be considered a first-time offense. God and country, however, saw it otherwise. Jeff knew it fairly quick, too, counting the years on his fingers. The limit had been raised to ten years between offenses.

Son of a bitch.

As before, as an attorney should be, Jeff was very casual about the whole thing. He'd seen it all so many times. It actual made me more comfortable, his laid-back attitude, and made me feel better just to be around him. He did not seem to share my perception that I was a total loser. Quite the opposite, he was very encouraging and, while recognizing the pain I was going through, also emoted a high level of confidence that if I would just keep my chin up, it would all be over soon. The sun would rise again.

As a people, we love to hate our lawyers. But in that deep, dark part of the night, when we really, really need them most, a good attorney, a guy like Jeff, is akin to a lover. In that time of need, they become the sweetest, most endeared person on the planet. No lawyer jokes apply.

I sat on a stiff plastic chair in the crowded hallway outside my appointed court room, waiting. Jeff seemed to be running late as the clock hit the hour. I knew he had forgotten me or worse, abandoned me altogether. But just as I imagined having to stand in front of the hang judge, naked and alone, sentenced to die by crucifixion, there he was, scurrying down the long corridor towards me, a bundle of files in his arms, a man on a mission.

All business, he barely had the mind to shake hands before "instructing" me to sit back down and wait for him. He would call me into the court room when needed.

"Holy crap, this is serious," I thought. "Like a television drama." With that, he disappeared behind the massive wood doors and I found myself, once again, sitting on that damn plastic chair in the hall where so many other abject loser criminals had sat before.

Not too long after that, he appeared once again, and didn't even stop as he pushed through the large doors and headed straight down the long corridor. He turned his head back and looked straight at me, motioning me with his finger to follow. Like a good puppy, I obeyed, lurching from my prison chair and catching up to his side, trying hard to match his urgent pace. "We have a problem," he said, no humor in his tone.

OK, those are not the words of confidence I wanted to hear. I was praying he would come out of the court room dancing, a broad smile across his face, and fist bump me. I was hoping the judge had a soft spot for drunken Irishmen or that the bumble-headed court administration had lost my file. But something else was unfolding here, and by his furrowed brow, I could tell whatever it was, it sure as hell was not in my favor.

He kept right on walking down the hallway toward the stairs. It felt like we were both trying to escape as quickly and quietly as possible without drawing too much attention to ourselves. "You have a warrant out for your arrest," he said. "We have to head over to the county jail right now and clear it up. Don't worry, it's a paperwork thing," he said, walking quickly and somehow seeming to pick up pace. "Evidently, somebody forgot to file something somewhere and it placed you in contempt of court."

I was speechless. Contempt of court? All I had tried to do, since the moment the handcuffs came off that drunken morning in jail, was be a good boy, pay my fines, show up, wear a stupid tie...I was being compliant, damn it. What more does this freaking system want of me? "But," he said, the lines creased hard on his forehead, "and this is the bad part...I don't know how long it will take to clear up. Could be immediately, or..." He stopped suddenly, almost leaving black shoe polish skid marks on the linoleum floor, "Or they might put you in jail again until it is."

Um, what?

Why Try to Fight? No matter what I did or how sorry I was, no matter if I was a nice guy or a bad guy, whether I wore a tie to court or not...it just didn't matter. I was in the system now and the system was an old, fat, blind giant that chewed on the bones of those who came too close to its rotten-toothed, ever-grinding, slobbering jaws. Contempt of court. Great, now what do I do?

We walked out of the courthouse, side-by-side, and made our way quietly now, a few blocks west to the county jail. Why the jail of all places? My mind was racing. This is a trap. I know it, it's just a trick to lure me back to jail, grab me by the collar and throw me in a stinky cell again. Why couldn't this be cleared up in a more comfortable, professional administration building somewhere. The city is filled with those places. But no, I have to go to the jail to plead my random case and not even my confident attorney is sure what the hell is going on or if I'm going to walk away from this.

We both stood in front of a small glassed window counter, an unemotional Sheriff on the opposite side. I think he was actually a zombie. I could see passed him, just over his shoulder, the caged widows and bars just beyond, faded green walls badly in need of paint, a world of brutality and filth, just waiting for me to step over the threshold where I would be seized, taken forcefully down dark corridors and disappear for years, maybe for life, forgotten, my files lost or shredded by some old woman, a state worker who loathed drunken Irishmen. I was going back to jail and I was going to die in there.

The dead-eyed sheriff and Jeff spoke for a few moments, shared several documents and figured it out. A good bit of stamping, stapling and the papers were returned. Jeff smiled at me. "Good to go," he said, as if he knew it all along. Truth is, Jeff had been almost as nervous me. The only difference was that he had not pissed his pants.

Like that morning I had been released from the drunk tank, it seemed a different world outside now. The sun was shining. The birds were singing, alive and beautiful. It could have been pouring down rain and I wouldn't have noticed. It felt so good all of a sudden to be a free man.

"There was a lame screw up. Paperwork. No big deal," Jeff confided. "I had to reschedule your court date, so we have to come back and do this all over again. Welcome to the justice system."

Several weeks later, when I finally did stand in front of the infamous Judge Roy McBean, heartless outlaw hang judge, he never even took notice of my new tie. The same paperwork he no doubt had seen countless times in his fifty-plus years sitting up there on his throne, still somehow managed to confused him.

He had several worker bees buzzing around him, the assistant District Attorney and a few other overpaid court workers, flipping the paperwork for him as he removed his glasses and rubbed his forehead. I think there was a small boy holding a plate of fruit, waiting to feed him grapes and sing him softly to sleep during his royal naptime. I don't think this old geezer enjoyed his job very much. It sure as hell didn't look that way to me. As a young man, he should have followed his heart instead and become a ski instructor in France.

Rather uninspired, he laid down my sentence, my fines, my penalties and restitution, handed the pile of papers to a little helper elf and motioned me away, out of his sight. That was it. All done. I was a hardened criminal and I was going to jail. So matter-of-fact. Again, McBean had seen it a million times, but I was not exactly used to standing there, several feet below a judge, a man looking down upon me, sending me to jail. Only this time it wasn't my imagination. This time it was real. I was going to go to jail.

A friend once told me, warned me actually, "Dude, you keep drinking like you do, and you're gonna end up in jail. And trust me," he continued, "you are not the kind of guy who will do well in jail…"

I'm not sure exactly what he meant by that last part, like maybe I was the kind of guy who cried at night and got raped in the shower, I don't know, but I didn't question him. I agreed whole-heartedly. I would not do well in jail.

———

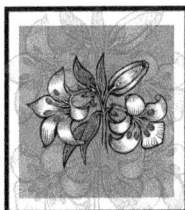

The Identity Crisis of
RICHARD TURNER

———

Is there such a thing as a mid-life crisis? I wonder. I've been told that I've been having one ever since I was twenty-years old, and strangely, I think it's true. Life has never been particularly clear with me who I am or what I'm supposed to be doing with myself.

Evidently, I'm not the only one. The fact that there is a quasi-clinical term for it, midlife crisis, suggests all too many people, if not every single person, both male and female, go through at least one period in their life in which they struggle with who they are, what they have accomplished, and possibly that they've wasted their life spending the majority of their days traveling down the wrong road. It's a horrible, gut-wrenching feeling.

Richard Turner was one of these people. Luckily, he figured it out even if it was in the latter half of his life. If you were to meet him and talk to him now, you might never imagine the man once served as the Deputy Attorney General for the California Department of Justice and as personal council to then Governor Ronald Reagan. Practicing law for over 40 years, he spent almost an entire lifetime sharpening his claws and, in his own words, would wake-up empty each day and ask himself, "So whose life am I going to destroy today?"

As an attorney, the bar doesn't get much higher than Richard had raised it. He was right up there at the top of the mountain. Wealthy, powerful, prestigious, for all intents and purposes he had accomplished a great deal. More than most. He was living the dream.

Or was he?

Somewhere in his 60's he found himself not much more than a soulless, empty shell of a man. Lots on the outside. Nothing on the inside. He told his wife one day, "I just can't do it anymore." With that, he packed up his car, tossed a few clothes in the back seat, a toothbrush and an old camera and told her, "I'm not sure when, but I will be back." He kissed her goodbye and set off down the road headed nowhere in particular. Maybe the real Richard was waiting out there somewhere.

Traveling well over 3,000 miles, when he returned over a month later, he quit law practice for good. During his time away, he found a particular interest in an old camera and the simple satisfaction of photographing all the beautiful and wonderful tiny bits of nature he found along the way. Beauty that had previously escaped his attention. Flowers, streams, birds, trees…all of these simple and quite ordinary objects suddenly appeared to him as living pieces of art, sculptures

*provided by God for those who would just stop and take notice.
And finally, Richard did.*

*He traded in his tailored pin-striped suit and classic red tie
for a pair of blue jeans, plaid shirt and beat-up old fishing cap.
There was very little now that escaped his eye through the
viewfinder of his new toy. With no goal in mind and no
particular sense of trying to accomplish anything, he just shot
one photo after another.*

*It was a close friend who, after seeing some of Richard's photos,
exclaimed, "These are really good, Richard. You should do
something with them. Make a book or something..."*

*So, that's exactly what he did. Only in the making of a book,
the muse paid a visit and he felt compelled to write something
to go along with it. Poetry of all things. Suddenly, this hard-as-
nails attorney turned into a budding flower himself, writing
poetry and photographing daffodils. It's quite possible President
Reagan and the majority of his legal associates talked about him
back at the law firm. Poor old Richard, he'd finally lost his
mind and went off the deep end.*

*In a sense, he did sort of go a bit whacky. I mean, who does
that? He spends his whole life carving people up for a living,
building his little empire one vicious lawsuit at a time, then
snaps and becomes a self-proclaimed poet, taking silly
photographs. Clearly, he needed the help of a good
psychotherapist. With one small exception; he was finally happy.*

*Out there on the open road, just him and that old camera,
Richard had found something indeed. He had found his true
calling. However long it had been calling his name, he finally
heard it and listened. And the answer changed the entire course
of the rest of his life. From attorney to artist, he slammed on the
brakes, spun a one-eighty in the middle of the street, and headed
off in the opposite direction.*

His book, "I Can't Always See My Path…But I Keep On Walking" became very popular, getting rave reviews from everyone who saw it. It then spawned the creation of a growing series of inspirational greeting cards as well, selling all over the country as fast as he could create them. Like a little boy, he grins and giggles now as he admits to the strange place he now finds himself, reflecting back on the cold world from which he narrowly escaped.

From a certain perspective, one might feel a bit sorry for Richard, regretting all the time he lost in chasing the wind and climbing the proverbial ladder of success. The truth is, however, viewed from a slightly different perspective, how fortunate he is, blessed you might say, that unlike so many others, he was somehow able to catch a glimpse of something greater, drop everything and reach out for it before it was too late.

Sadness and regret are not things that haunt Richard. Those are the emotions more deserved of the poor souls who never find their passion, or if they do, ignore it time and again, only to have it slip away, like water through their fingers, never realizing what they could have had if they just let go.

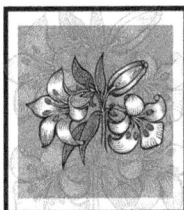

DRUNK SCHOOL FOR THE CRIMINALLY INSANE

JANUARY 19, 2017

I think this strange woman has lost her bloody mind. She is clearly certifiable. And she is my counselor.

Poor Barbara. Like so many well-meaning counselors in the lucrative industry of legally robbing drunk people, Barbara had paid her own dues along the way. Somehow, it became evident to her that it didn't take an I.Q. above 35 to qualify as a drunk-driving counselor, so she applied, became a counselor, and was eventually inducted into the Hall of Fame for deranged comedians.

A portion of my sentence handed down from the Judge's royal bench was a standard, court-mandated "Drunk School," a place for naughty people to go sit in the corner and stare at the wall. My penalty included a nice, long, eighteen-month exercise in learning how to control my temper and refusing to kill one of the counselors. Even if they did deserve it. In fact, I should quit referring to them as counselors. Honestly, it's not fair to them as it places far too much respect and responsibility on their shoulders and a position of intelligence they simply cannot attain. As they all seemed to be stamped from the same factory mold, let us simply refer to them as minions.

Barbara was the chief of the silly minions and boy did she love to make that point. She taught an education class that was nothing less than a sideshow circus. As her story had been told behind her back, she was an offender like all the rest of us. Only Barbara's story was a bit more colorful than most.

Driving stone, cold drunk one late night and trying to escape the police, she had taken a freeway off-ramp a little too fast and broken through the guard rail, sailing off the high embankment only to be saved by the hand of God, her car landing firmly in the top of a tree. And that's right where she was when the police arrived, high up in the branches, talking to herself.

At times, I simply could not believe what I had been subjected to and often looked around for hidden cameras, filming us, as though some sort of secret test on unfortunate lab rats. This woman would say things that made absolutely no sense. She would mumble and rant about God only knows what, shift her thoughts several times midstream, and continue right on, adding an exclamation point at the end of her sentence as thought that made it all legitimate. Perhaps she had seen a television evangelist or two who subscribed to the same approach.

People imprisoned in the class would watch her, waiting patiently for anything she blurted out that might remotely resemble just a tiny hint of organized communication, often glancing nervously at others in the class to see if they too were as confused. She was speaking in English, that much was established, but the words that came burbling out of her non-stop lips did not fit together in a reasonable fashion and made no intelligent or reasonable point whatsoever when combined. She was a human jigsaw puzzle created from the pieces of a thousand different puzzles. And for two solid hours, every week, this painful torture went on.

Luckily, there were to be only six of those particular education classes. I guess they had experimented prior to my attendance and six was the maximum any person could mentally endure before their brains self-combusted and ignited those sitting around them. My brain had not reached that level quite yet, but a decent portion of it had definitely melted beyond repair. Perhaps I would now also qualify for becoming a counselor, or minion, sorry.

Next on the agenda was Group Discussion in which roughly 20 people would gather in a room, pretending to be alive. There was a daily topic introduced along the lines that might be relevant to a group of seasoned alcoholics, but the discussion rarely, if ever, came anywhere close to touching on that subject. Instead, 95% of the inmates chose to tune out as best they could, scrutinize the tips of their shoes or the occasional fly on the window sill, while the other 1% blathered on about oil filters and the ingredients found in hot dogs, dominating the class with other such randomly interesting subjects, from the likelihood of whether or not the Kansas City Chiefs would trade Alex Smith at the end of the season and where he might end up, to the exact GPS location of a new or an old restaurant in town, how many times they had eaten there, and what was best to try on the menu.

Keep in mind, these subjects of discussion are not uninteresting in and of themselves, just not exactly relevant in the given situation. Especially when you don't really give two cents about any of it. Then it just plain hurts. Again, for two solid hours, every other week, for over a year, I had to listen to these two or three knuckleheads, people who live to hear themselves talk, and now with a captive audience.

The group leader, Ron, sat in the corner and chewed tobacco, waiting his turn to say something profound, but never finding the opportunity. There were times when I became convinced that he was merely a cardboard cut-out, propped there by the door way of the room to fool us and prevent us from leaving.

Finally, as part of my unjust sentence, there was a 15-minute actual counseling session that took place once every other week for a year as well. This is where you had the chance to sit down and discuss the difficulties in your life, the reasons you chose to kill the pain with alcohol, and how your troubles had not been resolved, merely increased as a result.

Or so I thought.

Imagine my horror upon arriving for my first counseling session only to discover that my revered counselor was none other than…Barbara.

"Oh, God, one more time…please help me."

Fortunately, these sessions were only to last fifteen pain-filled minutes. As should have been expected, however, they were anything but counseling. It was nothing more than a forced, face-to-face administration session, something that any normal human being could accomplish over a simple 2-minute telephone call, in which Barbara, however, consistently as confused and discombobulated as her bizarre communication skills, attempted to keep an "organized" file on each of her victims. It was like watching a chimpanzee try to fix a broken toaster. She would scribble random notes to herself, then in our next session, wonder who had scribbled them. Out loud and quite adamant, she spoke to herself often. Agreeing, then disagreeing. It didn't take me long to realize there were at least two people in her head. Likely many more.

She frightened me.

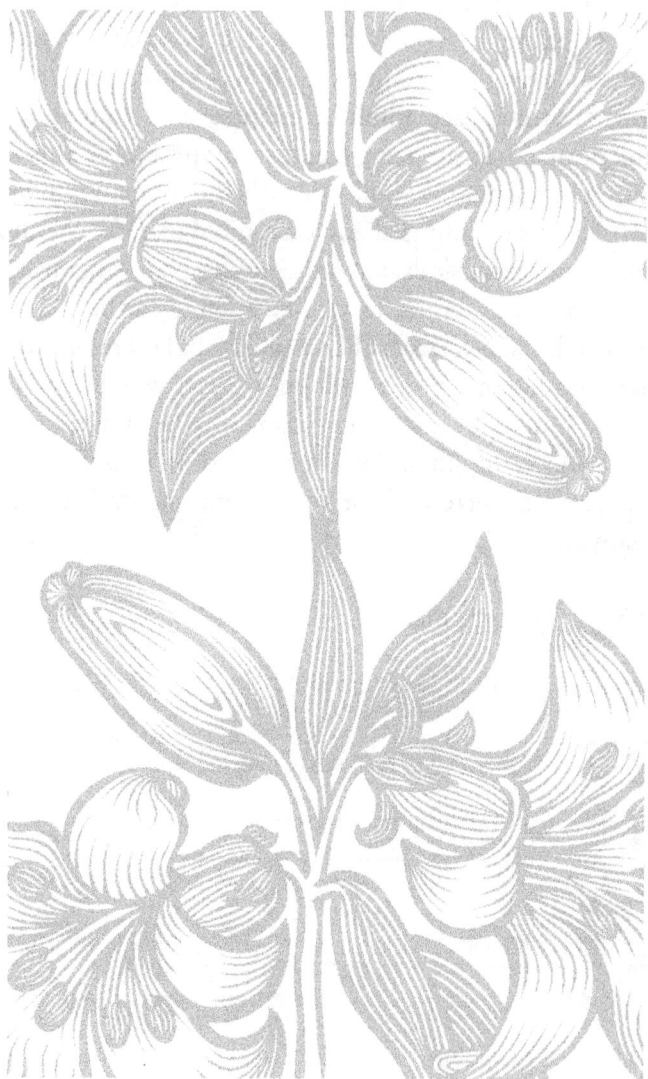

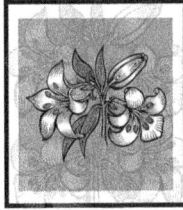

The Long and Twisted Road of
SABRINA CARTER

At just nineteen young years of age, Sabrina found herself sleeping under a bridge, alone in the cold, and pregnant. Born to a life filled with alcoholism, drug abuse and violence, she had never known a world without utter chaos and now, was about to bring another new life into that same dark place.

As a child, she vividly remembers her father chasing her mother through the house, screaming at her, beating her, threatening to kill her... while Sabrina, her sister, and younger brother hid outside, huddled together in the recesses of an old dog house. "I can still smell the rotting wood," she recalls, "and that horrible, sickening stench of wet dog hair."

After witnessing her father's death, a tragic hit and run accident, it is no wonder she too began abusing alcohol and drugs, even though she was shockingly only ten. By the time she managed to survive to the age of fifteen, she had become a seasoned drug dealer, selling whatever she could just to eat and make ends meet.

This was her life. This was all she knew.

And then…pregnancy. A baby. Born into a world of pain just like Sabrina's, continuing a seemingly never-ending cycle of poverty and pain.

Trying her best to care for her newborn child and quitting drugs in a frustrating attempt to clean up her life, she couldn't escape the people who kept dragging her back in. She became pregnant once again.

Despite somehow remaining clean and sober herself, with a roof over her head from a weekly motel room, she was reported and identified by Child Protective Services as risking the ongoing safety of her children. She lost both of them at once.

Even when it is in the very best interest of the children, it is painfully hard to imagine the torment a mother experiences in losing her children. The children too, not understanding what was happening, went through a living hell. While struggling desperately to put her life together, in the mere blink of an eye, her two babies vanished. She didn't know where they were or if she would ever see them again. They were simply gone.

She drifted, shelter to shelter, lost, empty, like a fallen leaf, blowing in the wind…until she landed upon the threshold of Saint John's Program for Real Change, an organization dedicated entirely to reaching struggling women stand on their own two feet and end the vicious cycle of poverty and addiction, not just for themselves, but for their children, and their children's children.

From the moment the Saint John's door opened, everything began to change. For the first time in her life, she was surrounded by people who loved her, helped her, and showed her how to stand on her own two feet. Education, therapy, job and life skills...things she never knew existed were al provided to her. "They gave me my life back," she whispers, tears streaming down her cheeks. "And then, the biggest miracle of all...they brought my children back to me. My babies...we are together again."

Sabrina graduated from Saint John's in 2016. Passing her high school GED, she landed a full-time job and found security in her very own apartment. "I changed from this broken, incomplete, frightened little girl...into a woman, independent, confident and blessed. I am a mother to my children. For the very first time... I am alive."

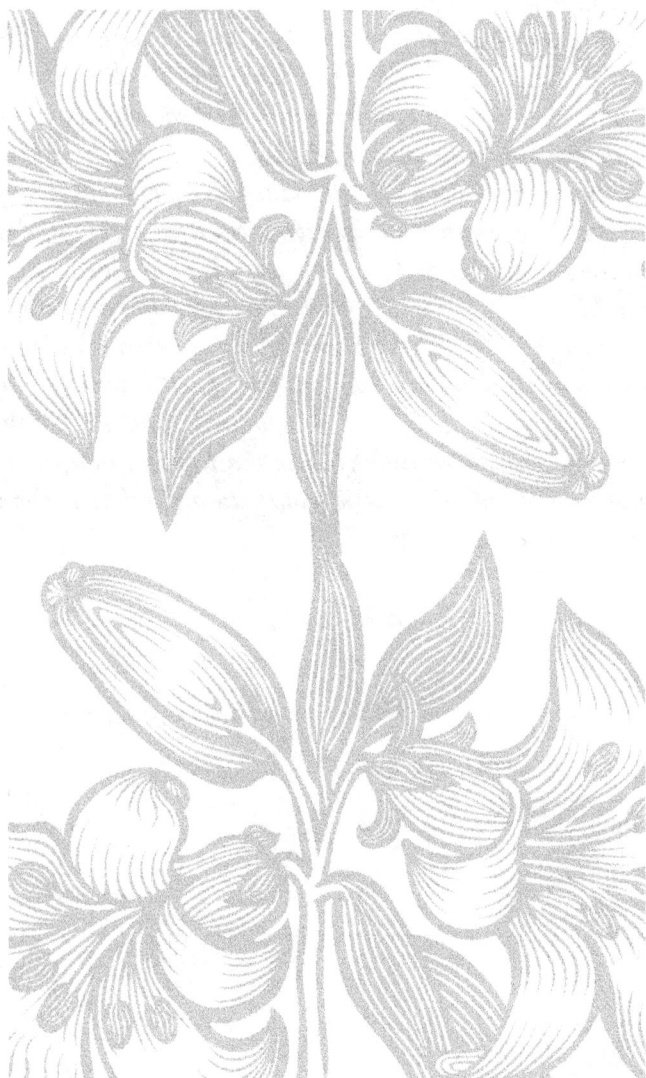

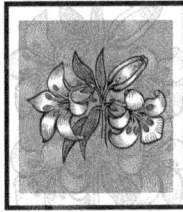

SERVING HARD TIME

———

FEBRUARY 24, 2017

———

I was suddenly faced with having to do something that has frightened me my whole life. Going to jail. The very thought of it, even now, is like a recurring nightmare. I never really thought it would happen. Not to me. Along this dirty, little road I've met quite a few tough guys who don't seem to think anything of it, a thorn in their side perhaps, but no big deal. For me, it was sheer agony.

The weeks and days leading up to the inevitable date were filled with anxiety and turmoil. My stomach was often tied in little knots. Call me a wimp, but I'm just not good at dealing with stuff like this.

The impending day finally arriving, my brother, John, stood by me, taking me and waiting with me, sitting in the parking lot in his car, talking, reminiscing old times, laughing, anything to ease the pain.

Eventually, however, the time came, and we had to part ways. I said good-bye, entered the decaying County Jail and "turned myself in." After that, the next series of events became a blur of non-human zombieness. A part of my brain clicked off and I felt as though I was watching myself in some chain-gang movie. *Shawshank Redemption*, previously one of my favorite films, came to mind. In fact, it felt a whole lot like *Shawshank*.

It literally took almost five hours for them to process me and a group of twenty other mass-murderers. As expected, they stripped us all naked and used a flashlight to examine areas of my body that nobody has a right to examine. Not even my doctor. Not like that. Standing in a line of naked men, proudly bending my posterior and other extremities for review, one of the guards actually had the nerve to say, "Come on, fellas…this is harder on us than it is on you." I actually laughed at that point. Before I could stop them, the words, "I don't think so!" blurted out of my mouth. I immediately regretted it, but the officer took my sarcasm as it was intended and simply smiled. I think he realized I was right.

I was given standard jail clothing, including a pair of dark grey underwear that, despite being too tight, had once been referred to as tidy whiteys. They'd lost their luster several years prior, having hugged the sweaty butts of ten thousand men. I somehow ignored this fact and kept moving.

By a little after 11:30 in the evening, we were marched single file through a series of large metal doors and out into the prison yard, a labyrinth of high, razor wire lined fences with barracks in every direction. Each cell block building was packed with men, leering out the windows at the newcomers, fresh meat, just like *Shawshank*. I hoped I could gather and maintain a small sense of courage and be *Andy Dufresne*, not the fat dude who cried at night and eventually got beat to death for it.

This is where it got even more difficult. We stood in the yard, given a mattress and two blankets. We were approached by representatives from specific ethnic groups who demanded to know where we belonged. I somehow managed to understand the game and mumbled something about being white. I guess it worked because the guy seemed satisfied with my answer.

We were marched once more into one of the barracks, inspected by all the other inmates, again, just like the movie, and ushered over to our pre-assigned bunks. As before, I was immediately accosted, approached by a short bald-headed guy with tattoos all over his body, including his face and asked point blank, his eyes inches from mine, "Are you Wood?"

"Am I what?" I asked as politely but firmly as possible.

"Are...you...Wood?" he asked again, a little harder, and slowly, as if I might be hard of hearing. Suspecting that he was asking the same information as that other emissary out in the yard, I offered the simple, rather obvious fact that I was white, to which he greatly relaxed his tone, and welcomed me with open arms. "Well, then you're Wood," he responded. All was well.

I had done my research. I had heard the stories. It took me a beat or two, but I quickly figured out that "Wood" was short for "Peckerwoods," a rather brutal white supremacy gang that has virtually taken over our nation's prisons. And sure enough, there I was, on top bunk #37, dead center in the middle of a murderous skinhead gang, bunking directly over the cell's gang leader.

I'll call him Ben, even though that's not his real name. He was a strange little man, like most of the other inmates in the barracks, always giggling and laughing at something that wasn't even remotely funny. More than disturbing, it was text book insanity.

Within a day or two of these bizarre fits, it dawned on me that this non-stop laughter was actually a form of communication, a pressure-relief valve that the men incorporated into their conversations to ease the stress of being caged up like a parakeet. They all gathered in groups and guffawed, full belly laughs, at the most random things; a broken shoelace or the color of the wall. It wasn't real. It was forced. If an actor in a movie laughed like that, it would be rejected outright by the director. "Cut! Take it again from the top. This time laugh like you mean it!" It drove me out of my skull.

Making it worse, there was a television somewhere, on full volume, tuned to some whacked shopping channel, until all hours of the night. I figured it was a devious plan to drive the inmates whacko and let them all kill each other.

By the time I made it up onto my bunk, I was exhausted and somehow actually managed to get a few hours' sleep that night. I know I did, because around 4:30 a loud buzzer woke me up and almost knocked me off the bunk, announcing that it was chow time.

Who the hell eats breakfast at 4:30 in the morning?

Once again, a long line of men, all dressed alike, rambled single-file through the blackness of the early morning prison yard toward the mess hall.

We were handed plastic trays and a single plastic spoon, then treated to the most amazing pile of dog crap I have ever witnessed, fully expected to eat it. Everybody sat at long metal tables, just like the movies portray, and were not allowed to talk to each other. People did, a word here, a whisper there, "pass the *Grey Poupon*," things like that, but for the most part, you shoveled the contents of your plate into your mouth as quickly as possible and hustled back off across the yard, by yourself this time, to crawl back into bed and hide.

The food, if you really can call it that, had to have been a cruel joke. Like an obnoxious reality television show, the guards likely bet on who would actually eat the slop. Void of anything resembling meat, vegetable, or fruit, it was a clotted pile of leftover dog vomit. I forced myself to try it, as over the days I grew increasingly hungry, but simply could not stomach it.

One obese gentleman, taking constant note that I was picking at my potato clumps, asked, "You gonna eat that?" I shook my head and he just as quickly reached across the table and slid my tray beside his and kept right on shoveling. Ah, how sweet. I'd made my first friend. For the five days I was at *Shawshank*, I existed mostly on shriveled oranges, badly bruised apples, and an occasional slice of wheat cardboard. Water, too. The water was actually quite delicious.

Naively mentioning the length of my stay there in Shangri La, five long, excruciating days, the other men referred to me, not without a smile and a good deal of laughter, as "Short Timer." As I came to learn, many of them had already been in there for years and were facing even more. Compared to most in there, I guess it appeared I was on vacation.

One afternoon, after the lunch fiasco had finished, we were allowed to head out into a distant yard, clumps of overgrown grass and mud holes, where a game of football ensued. I chose not to play, rather sit and watch as did many of the wiser old men. Football in prison is where men get to take out their vindictive angst against each other and the guards won't say a word. Broken bones and noses are not unheard of.

Shooting hoops by himself on an adjacent blacktop area, crumbled with age and lack of repair, was a young man with no shirt on and a belly that, no exaggerating, almost touched the ground. He was so fat and so proud of it, that he would grab chunks of his jelly gut with both hands and swing it back and forth, taunting onlookers in the sadistic hope that someone would make a distasteful comment and he could then smother them or beat them to death with his stomach.

Strangely, the more I looked at this kid, the more familiar he became. I never approached him, fearing for my life, but believe he was a kid named Johnny, whom I actually once taught in Bible class at a Baptist church over a thousand years before, way back, unstained by life, when we were both still saints. Everything about him, except the steady stream of foul language that poured from his flapping mouth, told me it was the same little boy. Only older and much, much heavier now. Angrier, too.

When I first entered the jail days before, during the processing, they had taken blood samples, blood pressure and other vitals. Hepatitis is a big deal in prison or at least they think it is. I remember the nurse looking up to me from her chair as she squeezed the little pressure pump, my arm turning purple, and in mutilated English asked if I had high blood pressure. "No, I don't think so," I responded. "Hmmm, ok," she responded, obviously disappointed, "because your pressure is a bit high."

Yeah, no kidding. I'm being tossed in jail and paraded around like a zoo animal and it surprised her that my blood pressure was a little high? Whatever.

That said, for insurance reasons I'm sure, not genuine concern, they decided I was older than most of the convicts and at risk of keeling over at any moment. They placed me in a group of other lucky individuals that got to visit the Nurse Practitioner every morning to document our declining health. I say lucky, because it actually was a nice break from lying on my bunk reading trash. As long as the sun was shining, I took the opportunity to stroll as slowly as possible across the yard to my "appointment," enjoying the leisurely excursion as best I could. Guards, way up in the center tower, kept an eye on me, but I had permission to be there, so I used it to my advantage.

I must say, after the second day, as difficult as it was eating and bunking in an insane asylum, the stress eased ever-so-slightly, and it became just a little easier. The thought crossed my mind that I would survive this and that if I could just manage, hold my breath a little longer, I might just make it. This was a major mental break-through as I had not had that thought until this point. Prior to that it had been entirely disastrous, doom and gloom crap stuffed in my head. The possibility that the sun would come out tomorrow was quite helpful.

My brother John came to visit me and, just like in all the movies, we sat on opposite sides of the bullet-proof glass from each other, speaking through ancient telephones. Only for some reason, our phones didn't work. It took begging the guard and convincing him we were not attempting to break out of jail to get them to push a stupid button on a console somewhere to allow us to actually speak to each other. But, when we did, it was so nice to hear his voice, although painful. We laughed at my situation. He said I looked every bit the part of a hardened criminal. I told him I was going to hunt him down and kill him if I ever got out.

Back in Cell Block 13, the incessant laughter continued throughout the day and well into the night. I slept as much as I could, at odd hours, trying to make the clock turn faster. Strange men, seemingly aliens from different parts of the galaxy, were packed like sardines in that barrack. And just like a school of brain-dead fish, they would swarm from one end of the building to the other, walking around in circles in what I later understood was a form of aerobic exercise, keeping their blood flowing. I suppose I would have joined them if I'd had to stay longer, but as it was, I kept to my top bunk, eyes glued to a paperback novel. I had the sneaking suspicion if I ever got down, even to use the rusted urinals, chances were good that I'd never make it back up on my mattress.

Speaking of exercise, I witnessed quite a few unique adaptations in the absence of weights or other traditional equipment. Several men shared a chair, used as something by which they would do push-ups. Makes sense, nobody in their right mind would want to get anywhere near that filthy floor. Another guy used his shower towel, threaded it through the bars on the window and, grabbing hold of either end, he planted his feet and leaned as far backwards as he could, then pulling himself forward toward the window, back and forth, in a type of reverse push-up. Pretty clever.

The whole place was an odd, random mixture of low-budget, do-it-yourself fitness enthusiasts and stark-raving mad comedians. Tattoos covered every inch of skin, toe-to-head. Even faces were not exempt. That same faded, blue ink seemed to flow throughout the jail and I feared I might wake up in the middle of the night to find it creeping up my legs, across my stomach, and toward my neck. OK, I'll be honest, I did consider getting a tattoo when I got out. I was a hardened criminal now, after all. Not the classic teardrop on my cheek, hammered out by some self-taught artist using a repurposed paper clip, ink made from salvaged tobacco spittle…no, something a bit more tasteful, perhaps a nice eagle in the clouds with a setting sun. Something pretty. Something professionally done.

On the fifth day, the day of my release, I was in a state of mixed joy and panic. Watching the clock, I knew approximately when they would call the names of the men who would be released that day. In the same breath, I had convinced myself that the system was so screwed up, my name would not be on that list and that they had somehow managed to lose my file and that I would rot in there. It's not a place you can politely approach a guard and complain.

That's a quick recipe for getting shot or at least pummeled with a night stick. *"Please sir, may I have another?"*

My name was eventually heard over the loud speaker, along with several others. A cheer of celebration and mockery rose from around the barracks as friends parted ways, cellmates who had laughed often together, pals who may never see each other again, hopefully, and those who had no idea why they were cheering except to pass the time away.

I jumped from my bunk and began gathering my mattress and blankets. You were mandated to bring what you had entered with or you weren't getting out. I was not about to disagree and scooped up my few items and tried to get the hell out of there as quickly as I could, when I was stopped, accosted by an eight-foot tall Cro-Magnon man.

The dude towered over me, a completely shaved head, except for his scraggly beard, covered in tattoos. While he appeared pleasant in his simple request for my blankets, his eyes held a secret desire to mutilate me if I blinked twice at him. I did not understand.

"Um…you want my blankets?"

"Hang tight," he said with a smile, grabbed them from my hands, and politely promised he would return. "I'll be right back." And with that he disappeared around the corner with both my blankets, leaving me standing there, the sheer sense of all-out panic returning.

The loud speaker crackled again. This time it was just my name they called. "Flanagan!" The guards were looking for me and I had just lost my freaking blankets, my one and only ticket out. In what seemed like an eternity, I waited. And waited some more. Then, when I was about to start crying, as promised, the great white giant returned with a gracious smile and thrust my now far lighter blankets back into my arms. "Thanks, man," he said. "I appreciate it."

He had torn each of my two blankets in half and refolded them, keeping the two stolen halves to create an additional blanket for himself. Pretty damn smart, except that he had done so against strict regulation, without my permission, and by default, had risked the very possibility of my freedom in the process.

What the hell was I supposed to do if I had gotten caught? Rat the biker out? He was a contract-killer for crying out loud. I don't think so.

My anger swelled, but my fear overruled it. On my way out into the yard, standing in front of the guard hut as they processed the men who were leaving, I made up the absolute best lie I could possibly think of under such duress. That damn voice in my head, the most irritating, condescending one, would not shut the hell up. It warned me, berated me, that if discovered carrying only two half-blankets, I was as good as dead.

I tried to look as calm, relaxed and pleasant as I could. I was one of the nice ones after all. A good man at heart. I would merely act surprised if busted, offer the God's-honest-truth, that was how the blankets had been given to me. I hadn't complained, despite the cold nights, because I was a good boy and only wished to remain compliant, grateful even, for any amount of comfort they'd seen fit to bestow upon me.

As it turned out, my fears were un-founded as I was bluntly directed to dump the dirty blankets in a large laundry bin along with all the other blankets. Nobody was counting the threads. Nobody paid any attention. Nobody cared. I could have been wearing a tuxedo, an orange curly wig, and a bright red clown nose and nobody would have batted an eye.

It took roughly six hours to process me when entering the jail and only about four to leave. In a final example of how screwed up they are in there, the guard shift changed right smack in the middle of my release. The fool-of-an-admin clerk who was managing my file failed on so many different levels to correctly transfer the information or provide any indication that my brother John was waiting out in front, right where he was supposed to be waiting, exactly where he told them he was waiting, obediently, where a big fat sign gave him no other choice but to wait…and yet, somehow, nobody knew anything about anything.

So, I sat, in a rancid, puke-smelling holding cell, and waited. And waited. And waited. Hours went by and finally, somebody noticed and, scratching their head, decided I had no transportation and should be placed back in the barracks.

I flipped out. "No way! My brother John is here, waiting for me," I said, in a tone that they either took seriously or as a potential threat. I got their attention and it wasn't necessarily good to do so. One of the guards looked at me with a strange, empty glare. "Let me check," he said, his hand resting precariously on his pistol, "Now sit down."

It took five short minutes to solve a problem that never existed in the first place. Faithfully, as I knew he would, just as we had previously planned a thousand times, my brother had been there all along. Waiting. They never admitted their asinine blunder. They never apologized. They didn't have to. I was, after all, a notorious criminal.

Seeing him, my brother, standing out front there, just beyond that massive wire fence as it rolled open, a doorway to freedom, was more comforting than words can express. I felt a rush of air pour out of me. I felt light-headed and weak at the knees. Tears were forming in the corners of my eyes. It was so damn good to see him. We hugged, one of those great, life-changing full-on bro hugs. My time in jail was served. Wimp, short-timer, old man, whatever...I had survived. It was over.

And my brother John had come to take me home!

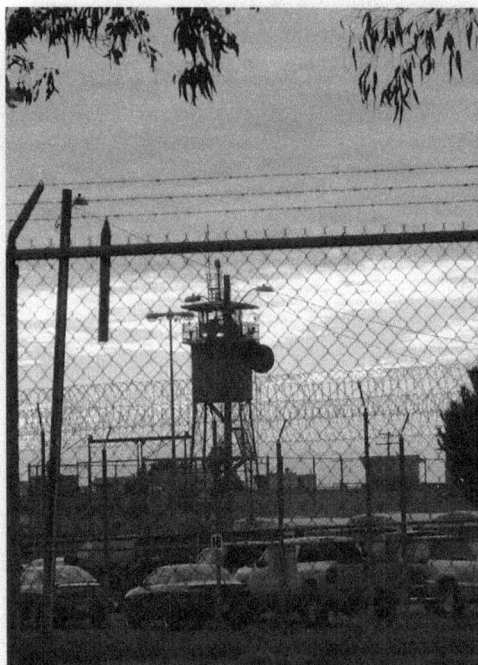

Rio Cosumnes Correctional Center, Elk Grove, California

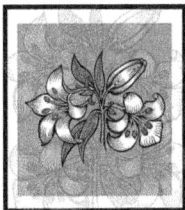

The Bizarre Dream of
BEN WRIGHT

I'm an official Peckerwood gang member now. In jail, I bunked directly above Ben Wright, the leader of the Peckerwoods. He was a short, stout guy, wearing his colors in numerous tattoos and a shaved head. The way he carried himself, the way he talked and laughed, he was a bull dog filled with spit and vinegar. But something he couldn't hide, was that there was a nice guy just underneath the surface. And just a little kid, too.

Other members of the gang would gather around his bunk, day and night. It was his office and where business was conducted, even if that business was simply telling lewd jokes or discussing their favorite female body parts.

One day, I happened to hear a conversation that was unordinary, unlike all the other previous senseless conversations. This one was about a strange dream.

Even though it was conveyed with much laughter, Ben relayed his bizarre dream because it was bothering him. I could see it clearly even if the others gathered 'round assumed he was just blathering on as usual.

I'm into dreams, the stranger the better, so I sat up and listened a little closer, trying not to be too obvious. Evidently, it was one of those dreams that are so vivid they stick with you well in to your waking hours.

He spoke of being at a wild party. It was his house and it was packed with all kinds of people, most of whom he didn't even know. The music was blaring, and everybody was laughing and having a great time. But for some reason, all he wanted to do, was get out of the house. As hard as he tried, however, there were too many people blocking his way, and inch by inch, he struggled to make his way toward the back door.

Finally, able to escape and step into the cold night air of the back yard, he closed the door behind him and stood out in the darkness alone.

It was then that he noticed a light turn on, from across the fence, coming from a neighbor's window. As he watched with increasing satisfaction, a young woman appeared in the window and began to get undressed. But she was no ordinary girl. She was, in fact, a girl Ben used to know when he was much younger, someone who, based on his comments, he had been "madly in love" with.

He approached the fence in an effort to climb over. He wanted to reach this girl, tap on the window and let her know he was there, that he still thought about her…but he couldn't. The fence was too high and no matter how hard he tried to climb it, he failed. He tried to get her attention, but he couldn't and after a time, she left the room and turned out the light, leaving Ben alone once more, in the back yard, in the dark.

Now tell me that's not an awesome dream. Tell me that isn't packed with symbolism and meaning. It's a classic dream and all I wanted to do was tell Ben what it meant. He assumed, as did all his gang members, that it was just a random, horny guy's dream about a Peeping Tom. I knew it was so much more.

But I was afraid. I was in jail surrounded by murderous thugs. I couldn't muster the courage to open my mouth, especially about something as freaky as dreams and their interpretations. I couldn't stop thinking about it, though.

I recalled the Biblical story of Joseph, a young Hebrew kid whose brothers were all jealous of him and sold him into slavery in Egypt. (Nice guys.) Like me, Joseph had a thing for dreams, too. Only Joseph wasn't shy about it. He would interpret dreams to anyone who cared to listen. It was because of this courage that he gained the ear of the Egyptian Pharaoh who had a particularly disturbing dream, and upon hearing the reputation of this kid in the local jail who might be able to bring meaning to his dream, the Pharaoh sent for Joseph.

Long story-short, Joseph was able to interpret the dream, save Egypt from seven years of blight and starvation, and earn himself a new title and all the wealth of Egypt. Not a bad gig.

Still, I'm no Joseph, and couldn't find the courage to speak up. Ben's little dream went uninterpreted. For the time being, anyway. So, moved by his dream, with what little courage I could find, I wrote Ben a letter a few days after I was released from jail and sent it to him. I knew, from hearing him read the letters written by his wife out loud to all who would listen, that my letter, too, would more than likely be shared among his homies. Only now, if they thought it was foolish faery garbage, they would not have the opportunity to stuff socks in my mouth and murder me in my sleep.

Evidently, pretending to be able to interpret dreams can actually get you in a whole lot of trouble when presented to the wrong crowd. It was Joseph's own brothers, after all, who sold him into slavery after becoming enraged by a stupid dream he unwittingly shared with them in which they would all eventually bow down to him someday. (Yeah...Um, oops.) His seeming arrogance sealed the deal for them to get rid of him forever. Forget the fact that it was true and would come to pass, Joseph had to pay a pretty high price to get there.

————

So, for Ben... this is what I shared.

The dream, his house, a wild party going on, packed with so many people whom he did not even know, making it almost impossible to move and preventing him from reaching the back door...

Hmmmm, is it just me, or is that pretty damn obvious?

So, Ben, can you think of anywhere in your life right now, where you might have a similar emotional feeling? Anything at all come to mind?

More often than not, in your dreams, a house, especially when it is your house, is a clear symbol for "your life." If this was true in Ben's case, was there any particular place or event in his life in which it was crowded, a large obnoxious party, packed with people he didn't even know, trapping him, and unable to escape? Duh… Jail, my friend. The loud party in his house was his current captivity in jail. It fit like a glove. (Not O.J.'s)

Continuing on, when he was finally able to maneuver his way through the wall of bodies and make his way out into the yard, it was cool and calm. Peaceful and quiet. So, where might that be? What might that mean? Again, using the symbolism of life and jail time, the freedom brought by the back yard was nothing more than his eventual release from jail. Someday in the near future, he was going to get out and the emotional feelings that would result would be identical to those in the dream of having escaped the bawdy party and breathing in the fresh, cool air of the quiet evening just outside the back door.

Then, in his dream, there comes this girl. Sexy as all get-out, too from his description. And someone he once knew, interestingly enough, and was quite in love with. (The love of his life and the girl of his dreams, you might say.) This was no ordinary sexually perverted dream, no, this was a symbol of his emotional attraction to this girl. He was crazy about her and had forgotten until that moment, seeing her there like that in the window.

So, tell me about that feeling, Ben. Is there anyone in your life right now, someone you may have been separated from, someone you actually love and would attempt to climb any fence just to reach? Who might that be? This is not a dream or a prophetic message simply encouraging you to go find that old girlfriend from your youth. She is merely a symbol, playing the role of someone in your life about whom you might feel the same way.

How about your wife? You know, that girl who writes you all those letters? The girl who hasn't forgotten you and is waiting out there for you to get out of jail? The one whom you really love deep down inside, but cover it up with jokes and macho laughter, pretending she is just your bitch? Yeah, what about her?

In my letter, I told Ben the meaning of his dream was pretty straightforward and simple. It wasn't me telling him what to do. It wasn't anybody but him telling himself what to do. This was a message from Ben to Ben. He just needed to understand it and listen. In no uncertain terms, disguised by symbolism perhaps, but very clear if you understand the language of the brain, he was telling himself... "When you get out of jail, and eventually you will, go find that girl (his wife) and climb that damn fence. Do whatever you have to do to reach her, hold onto her, and never, ever let her go. And above all, don't ever do anything to risk placing you back inside the party house. Of all places, that is clearly not where you want to be. Once in the peaceful freedom of your own back yard, realize what you have right in front of you, appreciate it, and never let it go.

Ben, you need to go apologize to your wife. Do whatever you need to do to save that relationship. She loves you and you love her. Stop all your drug-dealing bullshit, hanging with your street-thug home boys, and playing the part of the bad boy gang leader. It's time to grow up and invest in what really matters. And, coming straight out of your own brain, the love you have for your wife, is now the only thing that really matters. Screw that up, and more than likely, you'll get stuck right back in the middle of that very crowded party, one you don't even want to attend. Almost certainly, you will lose the "girl of your dreams" forever.

Well, wright or wrong, stupid or insightful, I don't know. But that's the letter I wrote to Ben. If he read it out loud to all the partiers in jail and they all had a good laugh at my expense, I'm cool with that. If he pretends my words are the ravings of a lunatic, that old man that bunked above him for just under a week, so be it. I know his dream had a deeper meaning, and it was his truth, not mine. I didn't make that seemingly random, bizarre dream up. He did.

I know, however, even if he does laugh it off in front of his supposed friends, it touched a deeper part of him. Nobody can come face-to-face with truth like that and not have it make an impact. He may choose to ignore it, sure, but I'm certain, after reading my letter, he was given a moment of clarity that he had never had before and one, that just might open the door to the back yard, a step toward his freedom and real meaning in his life.

I hope so. I truly hope so.

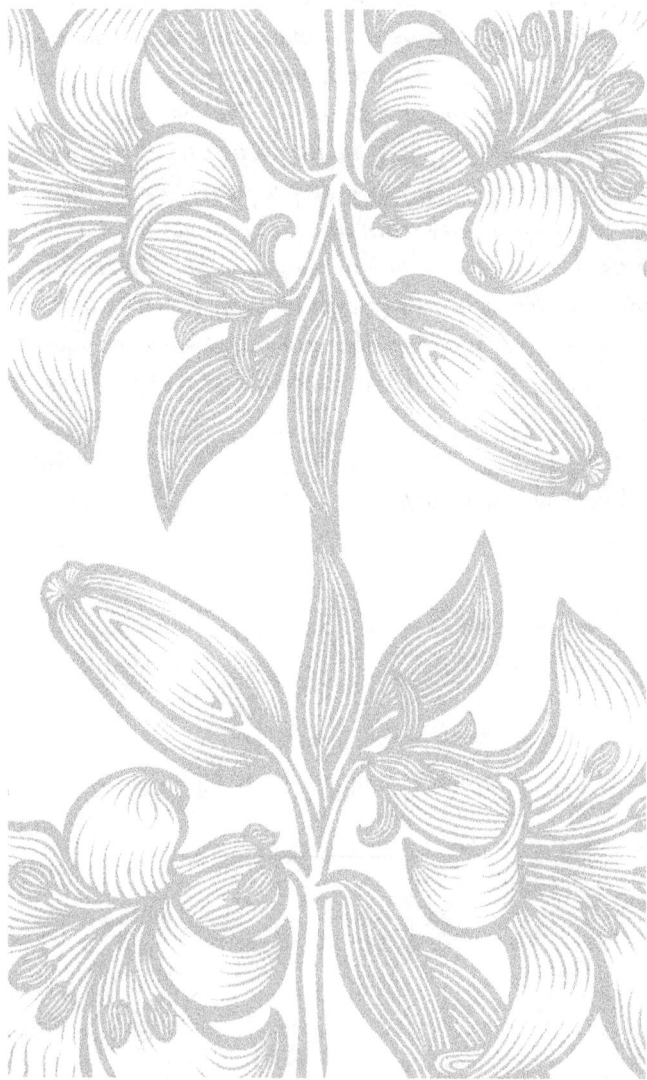

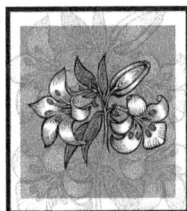

WORKIN' ON THE CHAIN GANG

———

MARCH 12, 2017

———

Standing in the center of an ancient historic graveyard, out of one hundred men gathered there in the cold, most were only half my age. I was clearly the old man in the group and way out of my element. Nobody cared. Nobody wanted to be there, old or young. Not even the sheriffs. I was just another body.

My "Community Work Project", as an additional penalty on my sentence, had been reduced to fifteen days for good behavior.

Wait...what?

Let me get this straight...I got sent to jail for five days for my bad behavior, then had ten days knocked off my community service for good behavior? I sure as hell wish somebody could have done a little more pushing of the pencil to jumble those figures a tad. I would have far preferred more time wandering through an old graveyard than sitting on a top bunk in a smelly prison filled with howling monkeys.

I was ordered to report to the *Sacramento City Cemetery*, a historic landmark filled with the remains and stories of ten thousand pioneers who somehow made their way all across the United States, fighting for their lives against angry natives, thieves, wild animals, and always sheer starvation....in search of gold.

All their names, men, women, and children, were left here, etched into the crumbling stones that marked their final resting place. In that sense, I found it rather cool being there. In a strange sense, I sort of liked it.

What I did not like, rather loathed, was the criminal element and the low-life way in which we were all treated. It's not that the presiding sheriffs did anything wrong, necessarily, just the ways in which they were required to do their job. They were, after all, having to deal with a motley gathering of convicted bums. No easy task.

We had to line up in rows, our feet touching a yellow dot painted on the asphalt. When we were all assembled, we would count off, raising our hand as we shouted out our individual number. Each time somebody would get it wrong, screw up their number, and force us to start all over. It was quite entertaining witnessing some idiot who had never learned how to count passed ten or that twenty-one immediately followed the number twenty.

We were frisked, making sure we had no cell phones, knives, guns or jack hammers in our pockets, then took our place in line. The whole process took about an hour, but that was one less hour we had to endure this slavery.

The guy next to me in the line smelled heavily of booze. Obviously, he had been drinking like a sailor on-leave the night before. He looked like he'd been sat on by an elephant's butt. And that rancid stench of vodka…the stuff was literally pouring out through his skin. No breath mint was going to help this poor sucker. If the guards caught wind of it, he would have been tossed in the back of an awaiting patrol car and hustled right back to jail. They don't suffer fools on the Chain Gang.

Somehow, he got away with it though. Everybody in line knew he was smashed, but lucky for him, the guards missed it. Maybe we all smelled that way to them.

There were always about three or four guards watching over and controlling the gang. Most of them treated us decent. A few didn't.

One officer in particular, Officer MaGee, stood above the rest. He was the commanding officer in charge of the others and, while he always maintained a cool sense of authority and order, stern and official, he never lost his humanity in the process. He always seemed to have a dry sense of humor lurking just beneath the surface, interacting with the men, treating them as humans, individuals, as though they had a chance at bettering themselves, not hopeless criminal scum destined to live behind bars. He was a good man and it showed.

One day, however, his boss showed up on the scene and it was more than evident, he wanted all of us to know who was really in charge. He took control like a drill sergeant and was hell-bent on finding some sort of wrong, somewhere, in someone, anything to exercise his supreme authority, which inevitably, he did.

At the end of our shift, at the hottest time of the day, the summer sun melting us all like hopeless chunks of butter, he refused to let us go. He penalized the entire group of men due to one man talking too loudly while in line. He said, very emphatically and by the book, "If you can't learn to follow orders, then you all will pay the price!" With that, even though our day was done, he sent us all back into the graveyard to pick weeds by hand.

I watched Officer MaGee through this whole ridiculous display. He rolled his eyes a few times, but bit his lip instead, allowing his boss to play big, bad, mean cop. MaGee would never have treated the men with such a kindergarten-style punishment. He didn't need to. He was better than that. He would simply have called out the offending man, the one with a voice too loud, told him to quiet down or go home for good. And that would have been the end of it. He was good at his job. The men respected him. I respected him.

I thought, that's what a good cop is like. Not some cartoon drill sergeant on an ego power trip, but a good man whose intent is actually to serve, protect, and help those men in his charge, lift them up, and put them back on the road to living a better life.

He has no idea, but Officer MaGee had a great impact on me and positively influenced my outlook on all peace officers.

I digress. Back to the graveyard.

On the first day of my community punishment, I made the huge mistake of raising my hand when asked if anyone of the newbies would volunteer for lawn mower duty. I should have known better, with only a few unwitting hands raised, that I'd blown it. The lawn mowers were old and had to be pushed by hand. Big and clunky, automatic drives long since broken, the mowers weighed a ton. Pushing those damn things around all day long, even a young man would have become exhausted. But I was no young man, and it just about killed me. At the end of the day, I had no earthly idea how I was going to make it through fourteen more days of that hell.

As it turns out, my amazing high level of intelligence to credit, I didn't have to.

By volunteering for mower service, I was unknowingly inducted into the all-envied and highly-respected *Power Crew.* (Gasoline-Powered Equipment.) Most of the guys had to labor all day long, standing in a single spot in the blazing sun, swinging a hoe at the dirt. But the *Power Crew*, no, we got to play with all the motorized toys; mowers, lawn-edgers, weed-eaters, and my ultimate selection…the mega-mighty leaf blower.

It was a tad heavy and a bit bulky, but once upon my back, it gave me a sense of self-mastery. Like a gun or a rocket-launcher, it has a trigger that allows you to increase the flow of air and blast the living hell out of anything in your path. Very satisfying.

In addition to the sheer fun of it, proclaiming myself as *Head Leaf Master of the Universe,* it allowed me the unique position and opportunity to stroll the entire cemetery, one end to the other, and back again. I was able to leisurely walk between the gravestones, often in the cool shade of the tall trees overhead.

I became increasingly fascinated by all these old, decaying stories of people who, like me, had once lived, struggled, raised families, built companies, and tried the very best to create a life worth living. These who were all dead now, most long-forgotten, as I too would be some day. It was not a sad thing, seeing all these stone grave markers, rather, inspiring in a strange sort of way. It was peaceful, interesting, and a provided an unexpected perspective I would never have had if not given the opportunity to move so slowly about the graveyard, investigating, imagining all these lives, these people, one story after the next, one headstone at a time.

Sometimes I would talk to them, these dead people. Greet them respectfully. "Hello, Mrs. Marianne Adams, Loving Wife of Jonathon Adams," I'd say. "I bet it's been quite some time since somebody said that to you." Ok, it's a bit weird, I admit, but it felt quite natural at the time. I have no idea if these souls could hear me or even cared if they did. It really wasn't about that. It wasn't an attempt to communicate with the dead. Nothing spooky, dark or twisted. It was more of an effort to clarify my own life by addressing these people who had once lived just like me. True, none of them had walked around a cemetery for weeks on end with a screaming wind machine attached to their backs, but we were otherwise very much the same, living our lives and doing the best that we could.

I became very familiar with the old cemetery. It had long ago ceased to be a spooky place for me, rather more the historic park, filled with ancient memories. There were so many people here, long since dead and gone. So many stories. How had they seen the world? What sort of dreams and ambitions did they have? Were they happy? Were they frustrated, like me, filled with the desire to be somebody? Did they feel like they were always being pushed back down in life, like the ocean waves, endlessly crashing against the shore, refusing to allow that gnarled piece of driftwood to leave the shore?

All these people, now lying here buried, they were very much like me. Perhaps they had made a mess of their lives as well. They had strived and struggled and repeatedly fallen on their faces. Some had made a name for themselves, indicated by their impressive gravestones. Most did not.

Of all those individuals now lying six feet beneath me, all were but a fallen leaf, blowing in the wind, initially missed by those close to them, but then within a short span of time, never to be remembered. All these people, they had walked, talked, worked, and dreamed. And now, they were gone.

It felt like a cruel joke, yet for the reality of it, for God to create a man, to instill within his heart a dream, and then, just as he is about to realize it, take it all away. But in my wanderings, grave after grave, I realized it wasn't so cruel after all, rather, it was my perspective that was cruel. I was looking for something up ahead, meaning and fulfillment, like a distant goal to be reached. I wanted life to give me something, a debt owed in return for all that I had given. If I was to struggle so much, life then, owed me. Didn't it?

But standing over all these people, it dawned on me, life had already paid its debt. Life had already given me the gift that it had to give, and long ago. I just never saw it. These people buried all around me, they could see it. Life had given me everything it possibly could. It had given me itself. I was alive.

That simple thought struck me and stayed with me as I continued my stroll, blowing the leaves from one side to the other. Life was not about getting somewhere or attaining something. Life was about living, being alive, breathing, smiling and experiencing a single moment, the time I was given right then, standing in a cemetery with a giant leaf blower strapped to my back.

I smiled.

If the sheriffs guarding the chain gang had noticed me, the sole wanderer, standing there alone, grinning like I was, they more than likely would have assumed I'd been drinking. But for the first time in a long time, I hadn't. There in the middle of an ancient graveyard, listening to the whispers of the kindly deceased, I had found a very simple answer.

And it made me very happy.

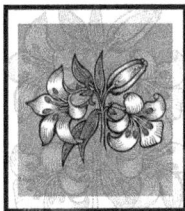

Nobody Really Remembers
MR. ANDREW ROSS

1830 - 1901

As I wandered among the gravestones…story after story, hidden deep beneath the ground, subtle hints etched in granite, eaten away by time, now covered in moss… I became drawn to one family tomb in particular.

— A. ROSS. —

Their gravestones indicated that the entire family of A. Ross was resting there as well, including his wife Catherine and their four children; Caroline, Pauline, William, and Katie. They had been lying there now, for so long. How many people stopped by to remember them? In the last hundred years, how many people had stopped and bid them hello? I did, finally. I took a moment and quietly, respectfully said hello as I tidied up their grave site.

But who was this man, his family, and what was their story? Where did he come from and how did he come to be here now? Surely, here lay a man who had seen life. But how? And how had it treated him?

Research showed very little. Even Google drew a blank. It was almost as if history made quite an effort to erase any trace of him. A man, who lived and died, got married and had a family, had all but disappeared of the face of the earth. I simply couldn't sit well with that. So, I kept digging, finding tiny bits and pieces, ship's logs, death certificates, marriage and business licenses...slowly putting the pieces of a puzzle together that eventually formed a clearer picture of a man that I now find, rather incredible.

One tiny article, hidden in an old newspaper clipping stated, "One of Sacramento's best-known businessmen... No man has a higher reputation for honesty and integrity than Mr. Ross, and he enjoys the confidence and esteem of the community..."

One of Sacramento's best-know business men... Really? Is that right? Why then did nobody seem to know a damn thing about him? Why was it so difficult to find almost any mention of his name? If he was one of the best-known business men, how had he so quickly been forgotten?

There was a story here, I knew it, and I simply couldn't let it die, buried and forgotten alongside this man. So, crude graveyard jokes aside, I kept digging.

————

Born in Aschbach, Bavaria in 1830, Andrew Ross lost his mother by the time he was 2-years old. That pretty much suggests he never knew her. What he did know was his stern father, George Ross, butcher by day, hotel-keeper by night. Working two jobs and trying to single-handedly take care of the children, a screaming baby included, I imagine life had to be a bit difficult for the Ross family.

By the age of fourteen, Andrew had sufficient schooling to call it quits and enter the butcher trade, working with his father until the seductive call-to-adventure repeatedly whispered his name.

In the year 1849, packing a single bag, he threw it over his shoulder and said goodbye to Germany forever, embarking from the port in Le Havre, France aboard a sailing ship bound for New York. Twenty-eight days at sea, just under a month, he stood on the deck of a ship, looking out over a vast ocean of blue nothingness, dreaming about what lay in front of him. He was filled with enthusiasm, ambition, and unbridled anticipation as, wave after salty wave, he drew closer to his destiny in the new world.

Barely a man, he was just 19 years old now. And like most men his age (identical to me), he stumbled around trying to figure out who he was, how to make ends meet, and what in the world he was supposed to do next. He hopped from around Milwaukee to Wisconsin, then to St. Louis for several years, cutting up chunks of meat and saving his nickels, while that old familiar voice of the siren, quietly calling his name. Only this time, with the irresistible lure of gold.

Likely, sitting around a tavern table with two of his drinking buddies over a pint of warm German ale, the decision was made to pack up once more and turn their faces west, toward the land where simple men were striking it rich and making vast fortunes. Danger be damned, Andrew was not about to be held back by the threats which had ended the lives of thousands of other hopeful immigrants. Thus, in the early Spring of 1853, now 23 years old, he defied the odds and set his feet toward California.

Something happened along the trail, what is not exactly clear, halfway through their journey in Salt Lake City, Utah. For there, he is known to have rested up for two weeks, then purchasing two ponies, and leaving his companions, he set out alone for the remainder of his journey. What ever happened to the other two men is anyone's guess. Perhaps the Mormon missionaries got to them. (Not a far-fetched suggestion.) For two men who had been sleeping in the dirt together for months on end, the lure of multiple wives was likely more seductive than gold. Not for Andrew, though. He could not be hindered.

Somehow, four months later, miraculously if you ask me, the naive kid actually made it. Sheer German determination or something. Thinking about it, he no doubt encountered all there was to encounter out there. It was the wild west, filled with pissed-off natives who hated young German butchers, almost no grocery stores, McDonald's or Starbuck's, and mean, hungry, lion, tigers, and bears... and yet, he survived it all.

I get upset and cranky when I have to work on the occasional weekend, but this guy, holy crap...he rode a horse across the entire country so he could buy some old rusty shovel and dig for rocks. Which is exactly what he did.

In the summer of 1854, Hangtown, California (now Placerville) witnessed a young man making his way down the mountainside to stake his claim. And yes, there's a reason they named the place with such a dainty title. Most never made it back to civilization. If they didn't get lost forever in the woods or eaten by Bigfoot, more men found the end of the rope than they did gold. It was a fool's errand, to be sure.

Out in the middle of nowhere, seven days a week, you work your sweaty butt to the tailbone, find a couple of microscopic golden pebbles, just enough to buy a gallon of whiskey to ease the pain, and maybe, help you believe what you're doing with your life makes good sense, then get into a fistfight with an Irishman who is actually more drunk than you, wake up with no memory of who you kissed or who you killed, and end up dangling from a rope for both.

Welcome to California, you stupid idiot.

Evidently, however, Mr. Ross was not as thick in the head as most. It took him less than a year to realize it was far easier to hack a pig to pieces than using a pick ax to smash rocks. He knew from experience, there was also more money is carving up a good steak than the few measly pieces of gold he may find. Sure, some guys got lucky and pulled the eight-pound gold cannon balls out of the ground. But most men, got nothing. Even those who did strike it rich, got a quick bullet in the forehead, their gold stolen, yanked from their dirty hands before they even hit the ground. Thus, Andrew set his sight on wearing slightly cleaner clothes and living the upright and ethical life of a city business man. Quickly landing a job at the local butcher's shop, he soon opened his own shop on 7th Street, just between H and I Streets.

I found this obscure little detail rather amusing, in that my own shop, a modern advertising agency, also sits on 7th Street, not a block away from this man whom I never knew. Like him, I too had become a city business man with a dream. How many other ambitions did we have in common?

The building in which my offices reside is the Pioneer Building, a historic landmark, originally a bunk and bath house for those filthy miners coming in out of the mountains to cash in their findings. Some believe it was more than likely a house of ill repute. In those days, men with gold in their pockets and the naughty girls who wanted it, seem to have gone hand-in-hand. It's quite possible that the esteemed Mr. A. Ross might have even paid a visit or two to my old building. Maybe even stood where I have stood and looked out the same windows. Maybe.

April 15, 1858 he met and married Catherine Faber, a good German girl from the old country. How could he resist? Not much is known or could be found about her at all, other than she possibly had a pension for raw meat and the men who carved it. She and her children are buried right next to Andrew now. But back then, it was all singing birds, fresh flowers and smelly sausages. Life was good for the Ross family, yielding four children, a healthy, well-respected business, and living life the best they could until the turn of the century in 1901.

And that's pretty much the end of the story for A. Ross. Not much else is recorded about this rather ambitious, brave and industrious man, with the exception of the fact that he died immediately, after he fell down and broke his neck. (Crazy 71-year-old.) After that, a deep hole was dug in the ground for him, he was covered up, then largely forgotten.

His wife Catherine, well evidently, she loved and missed him so much, she literally just keeled over only months after he had gone. "General Apoplexy" they called it back then, meaning some sort of internal hemorrhage, a burst blood vessel, a severe migraine, who knows. Almost nothing has been written about her. Missing her man, she just up and died.

———

Each weekend in the summer of 2017, I blew leaves, sticks and debris from the gravesite of Andrew Ross and that of his whole family. With no idea who this man had been, the challenges he had faced in life, what he had or had not accomplished, I kept his only remaining memory clean and tidy. I know his story now, or at least, have glimpsed it. I have a general idea of who this man was, what he was made of, and the life he struggled to live. I can only imagine the trials he faced, the burdens he carried, and the steep, unclimbable mountains he attempted. I have nothing if not the utmost respect for this man I never knew.

Now, with well over one hundred years gone by, I for one, remember Mr. Andrew Ross.

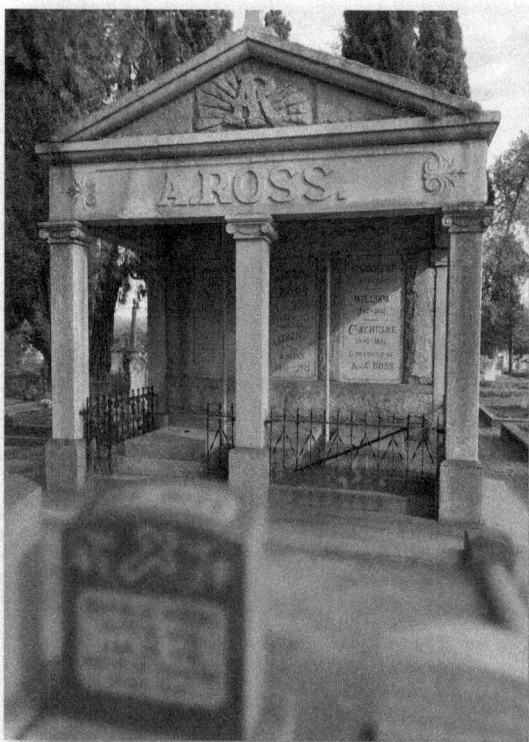

The only remaining memory of A. Ross, wife Catherine Ross,
and their children — Sacramento Historical Cemetery

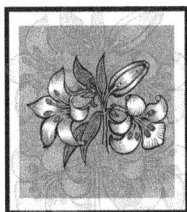

BOOM. BOOM.
OUT GO THE LIGHTS

———

APRIL 5, 2017

———

When life tosses a hand grenade in your lap, there's not a whole lot you can do about it. One of my business partners, John Hutchison, suffered a severe stroke, and just like that, the bomb exploded.

John and I had been friends since the early days when we were both in our twenties. Somewhere along the road, we lost sight of each other, both busy about building our empires, but somehow managed to reconnect, dream up a big dream, and decided to build a chain of automotive repair shops of all things. It was a strange combination of being in the right place at the right time (or wrong time), combined with the right idea and two capable friends. We came up with *Red Rocket Auto Tech* as a result. And between the two of us, it thrived, becoming a cool little shop.

Then, after seven years, when it came time to open our second location, we ran up the old credit line with the eager bank and made our castle walls taller. But just as the last stone was cemented into place, the wall came crumbling down, stone by stone, all the way to the ground.

John's stroke took him out of the picture completely. He was the driver who held the reigns. He managed the day-to-day operations, and without him, the shop didn't work the way it was supposed to. Service began to slide, pissing customers off, having to bring their cars back time and again for a simple repair that should have been fixed the first time.

We started losing money. Then, the floors stopped getting swept. After a day of greasy repairs, tools were left tossed to the side, buckets of oil, and broken engine parts were stacked in the corners until those corners had corners themselves. The lights in the parking lot sign went dead, and money being tight, it was decided to hold off replacing them. The once bright red awning that hung over the front entry, had faded now to a pale pink. The beautiful dream we had envisioned such a short time ago, was already dying.

Sometimes, life's difficulties bring out the best in people. The challenges they face serve as a test, like iron forged in the fire, making them stronger and better than before. But that is not always the case.

With John, the fire brought out his demons. He gave them the keys to his house and abandoned it, turning inward, dark and remorseful. He had always been a bit of a jerk, but now, faced with the lack of ability to even put a sentence together, he turned into a complete ass. I'm not throwing rocks here. It's just true.

I've known men who have literally lost their legs only to rise again, becoming great leaders, even motivational speakers, sharing words of inspiration and hope to others. I've seen homeless women who lived each day only to face the biting winter cold, near starvation, living underneath a bridge, somehow pull themselves back up and go on to serve and help others still out there on the streets. John, as it turns out, just wasn't one of these.

Pain and impossible difficulties have a different effect on different people. I suppose there still lies the possibility that John is not done with his trial. Perhaps he is still in the middle of his journey. I hope so. For his welfare, I sure hope so.

But as it stood, at the time of this writing, John was gone. He had given me the proverbial middle finger and told me to leave him alone. And so, I did. Knowing very little about the day-to-day operations of the business, I was left to shut it down, deal with angry creditors, attorneys, landlords who had not been paid their rent, and a whole line of people who wanted money. My dream suddenly turned into a nightmare and I was not going to be able to wake up and shake it off. I had to deal with it, and now, deal with it all alone.

So, while I was experiencing my own little tragedy, one of great immediate financial loss, including the inevitable loss of the fortunes yet to be realized, a strange experience began to unfold right along with it. Despite my rapid pulse and strained anxieties, I was not drinking. I had not, as I surely would have not so long before, turned to a friendly, soothing cocktail to anesthetize the pain. This was new.

I had the bizarre clarity to take a step back and notice it. Maybe I was making progress after all. If I could get through this fiasco, my business exploding, pelting me with shrapnel… I could do most anything. And, if I could actually get through it without booze, well then, I had changed indeed.

Then the thought occurred to me; what if this too, this twisted disaster I was facing, was a gift as well, strategic and well-thought out, by a power far greater and smarter than me? Someone who had the ability to stand above it all and see the bigger picture? Like the entire disgusting and humiliating DUI experience I was in, after reaching out and asking God for help, it came in a way I would never have chosen for myself. Not in a million, bazillion years. And yet, as a result, I was changing. Just as I had asked.

Only now, with a dream crumbling through my fingers, how was I supposed to pick up the pieces and move on? Unless, this was all part of it, the help I asked for. Given a certain perspective, maybe I was not finished with the pain that would change me.

That gave me a small sense of renewed strength. If it was all part of a divine plan, one that I did not have to control, then I could endure it. Even if it wasn't, the fact that I could not control it, whatever it was or whatever it would be, also provided a sense of unusual peace. Just a little. Enough to breath and keep walking forward.

The moral of the story here, I think, is that with a cocktail or two, I would have felt very little of this. I certainly would not have had that simple moment of realization. They talk about alcohol "masking the pain," and it sure as hell does. That's the beauty of it. That's why it's so damn attractive. Nobody wants to feel the pain. The other side of the coin, however, is that's also why it is so destructive. It prevents us from growing, from hearing, from seeing. It denies us clarity in the painful moments in which we need it most.

In a journal I kept when much younger, I scribbled a note to myself, not realizing at the time how prophetic it would be thirty years later.

"Pain is God's favorite tool and the first step towards helping a man to change."

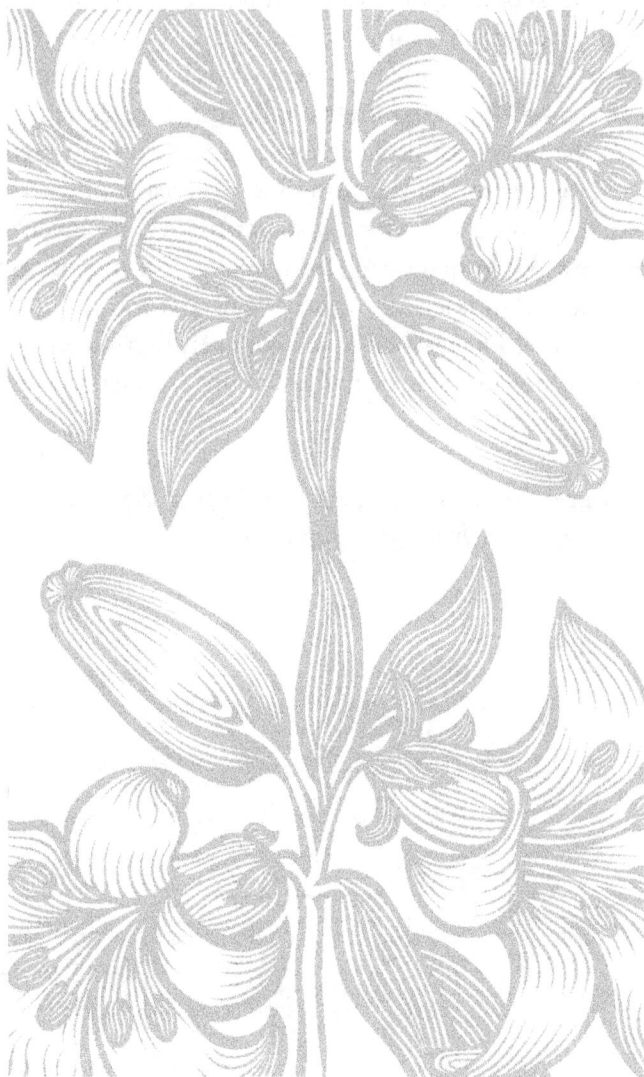

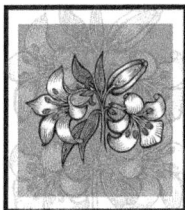

The last legal trial of

WILLIAM A. GETT

1864 - 1920

This is one of those sad stories that is as ironic as they come.
It starts out, the good life, and when things are bright and
cheery, looking up and enjoying the fruits of your labor, along
comes that old proverbial bus and kills you dead.

I first had the pleasure of meeting Mr. William Gett, his
gravestone rather, during the shooting of "My Sweet Suicide,"
an independent movie I wrote and directed in the summer of
1996. It was there that a certain romantic scene took place,

William's gravestone center stage, and as it played out, became the image used on theater promotional posters and eventually the DVD cover as well. I had no idea at the time who this gravestone belonged to, nor the story of the man lying beneath the feet of my entire film crew.

Twenty years later, I had the pleasure of blowing leaves from the same gravestone, now a criminal serving my sentence. Little did I know that Mr. Gett was, long ago, an attorney in my same town. Nor did I know, like me, he was born and raised in Sacramento. Further still, I could not have known his office was right downtown, spitting distance from mine. And finally, stranger still, the place he died so suddenly while walking to work, was a place I walk every single day.

But I digress.

Born in 1864, the son of a gold-digging 49er, William Gett was for all intents and purposes, a gifted, kind and incredibly respected man, honored by his clients, peers, and the local judiciary as having "a large circle of friends and one of the most popular members of society..." Wow. I wouldn't mind if somebody said that about me some day. An upstanding citizen and successful attorney, he had a good life.

At the age of 28, an old man in those times, he asked Ms. Ema Sweeney to be his wife. She turned out to be quite the industrious socialite herself, elected as Grand Vice President for the Native Daughters of the Golden West, a political activist and hostess of some rather erudite dinner parties according to the local newspapers. Evidently, young Ema was quite a windstorm. It is unclear whether the two young lovers ever had any children. Perhaps they were both too busy with their community efforts to concern themselves with such things, never imagining that fate would rip them apart, giving them no chance to further their namesake.

On September 28, 1920, William was strolling along I Street in downtown, Sacramento. Minding his own business as he had every day for years, he made his way toward the corner of 7ᵗʰ Street. Taking note of a certain street car that had suddenly stopped, slamming on its screeching brakes right in the middle of the intersection, he never knew what hit him next.

Perhaps the squealing metal of the train was just loud enough to prevent him from hearing the whistle blow from the oncoming truck. M. Lockett and R.E. Connell were driving east on I street, carrying a four-ton load in their company's two-ton truck. (It wasn't recorded what they were transporting. Possibly watermelons.) When the fateful street car suddenly came to an abrupt stop directly in their path, they "had no choice," as later stated in court, "than to yank the steering wheel sharply to the right…" Unfortunately, for him, that's precisely where William Gett was standing.

Court records show that Mr. Gett did not seem to hear or respond when the driver of the truck yelled at him to get out of the way. (Bummer.) No wonder he didn't move as he was struck hard by the overloaded truck's right front fender. It knocked him to the pavement like a bowling pin. Continuing in their effort to avoid the train, the truck then dragged poor Mr. Gett under its back wheel for "some distance," as the newspaper stated, "then… ran over him completely." The hopelessly out-of-control truck then slammed into the back side of the train anyway.

As the dust cleared, Mr. William A. Gett lay in the middle of the street, his back severely broken, only to die two extremely painful hours later. Holy crap! Here's this quintessential nice guy, minding his own business, taking a leisurely stroll, when… Bam! Lights out!

Goodbye, Mr. Gett. It was nice knowing you.

Ema Gett, yeah, she was not happy, to say the least. In fact, based on the little information I could find, she sort of flipped her turn-of-the-century bonnet. Evidently inspired by her husband's litigious line of work, she wanted blood, dragging both men in the truck, their company, as well as PG&E, owners of the street car, into a long, drawn-out court battle demanding a whopping sum of $200,000.

Heyy, that was a lot of money in 1920. Whether she ever got it or not is unknown, but based on court documents, it appears she fought tooth and nail for it. Her claim was that both parties were negligent in their responsibilities and their decisions resulting in the brutal death of her husband.

Nine years later, in 1929, Ema also died, for reasons unknown. Both are buried now in the peaceful cemetery in which I both made a movie and served my sentence. I had no idea who these two people were, how they had lived, succeeded, struggled and died. I don't know if they had dreams of starting a family, or political ambitions for the White House. All I know is that they were once alive and now, both dead and gone.

Finding any scrap of details about these two lovers was almost fruitless. And this lack, of one of the most prominent couples of the time, how can this be? The only available bits and pieces strung together begin to tell their story, but certainly nothing of the real people. There is no hint at who they really were, or what they longed for in life. Were they happy? Were they fulfilled? Did they accomplish what they were placed on earth for? Who can say? They are long gone now. Completely forgotten.

So, is this a sad ending? I'm not sure, really. It depends upon your given perspective. From one point of view, it could be argued that it is nothing less than a tragic ending. An innocent man plowed over in the street, his back snapped like a twig, his wife fighting furiously for justice, only to wear out, exhausted and empty, dying herself. Or, perhaps, is it just the way the wind blows and the story of life itself, neither fair nor unfair. We are to live our lives as best we can, but we never truly know when death approaches or will call out our name. We can't fight that. We can't be angry at the seeming injustice of it. It simply is what it is. Life. Then death.

For me, I choose to see their lives as happy. Well-lived. The two of them together, they did great things, even if it was a simple dinner party for their friends now and then. They loved each other, I assume, and certainly that was meaningful. In addition, almost 100 years after they breathed their last, some strange guy, a filmmaker and convicted criminal, stood by their grave, thinking about them, venturing to honor both.

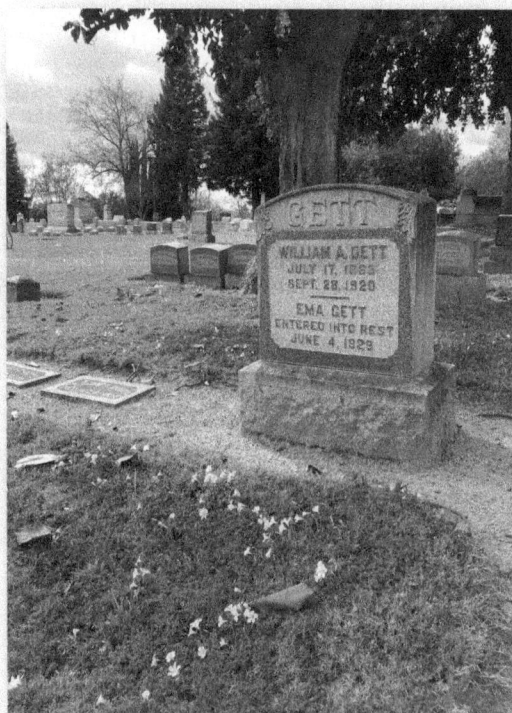

William and Ema Gett. Rest in Peace.
Sacramento Historic Cemetery

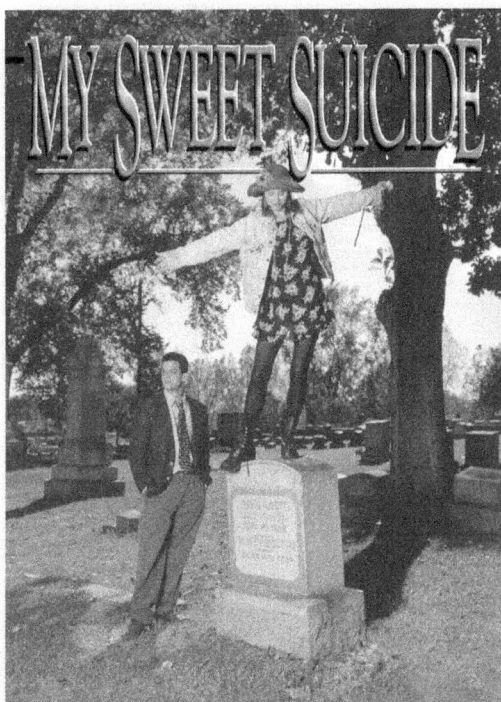

Movie Poster for my independent film:
My Sweet Suicide

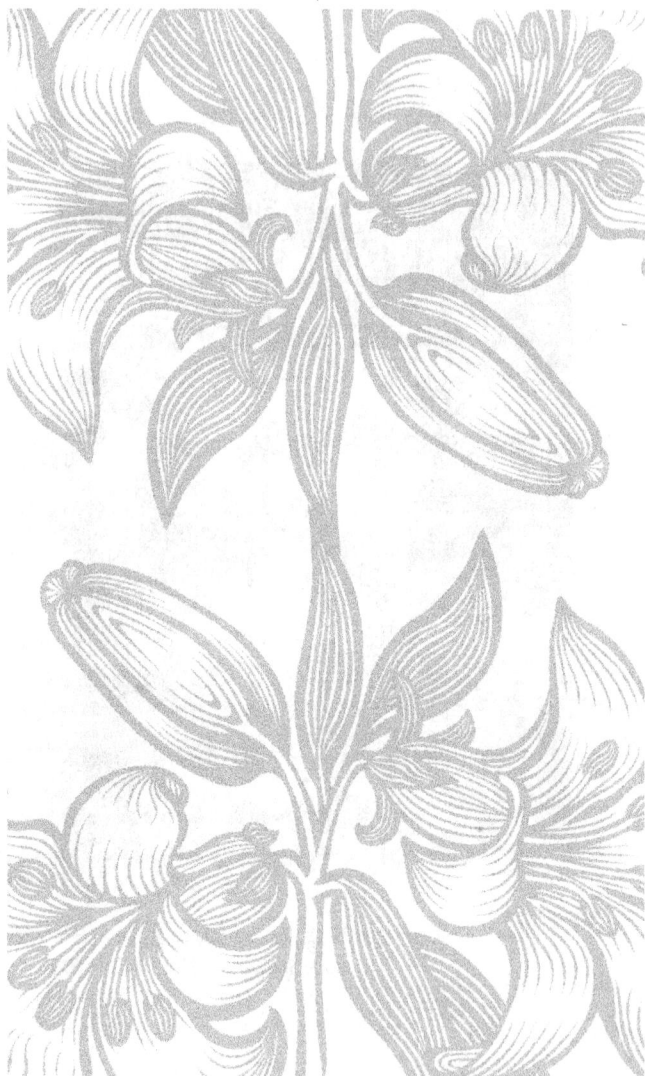

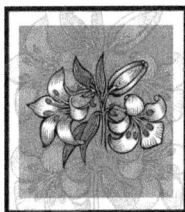

A CROSS-DRESSER'S NIGHTMARE

MAY 4, 2017

I believe in dreams. Not so much from a prophetic perspective, as in, "This weird or horrible thing is going to happen…" but in a more creative, psychological approach, as if dreams were our mind's way of holding up a mirror for us to see ourselves from a different perspective. Not the real you, rather just a reflection.

I've got to believe this, otherwise, the dream I had the other night means I'm in big trouble. Extremely vivid and filled with symbolism, it was, in a word, outrageous. It was so strange, that when I woke, I was really confused. The intensity and ridiculousness of the dream, however, and my respect and understanding that dreams don't mean what they appear, rather reflect another story, I knew there was a lot of meaning packed into it.

In the dream, I was sitting behind the steering wheel of a car, driving down the road. As I have come to know about myself, as it is for many people, this is a symbol of my life. My wife dreams about a home with many hidden rooms, I dream about driving a car. It's my symbol. Everybody's got one.

Anyway, sitting next to me was this rather sleazy consultant, a professional wardrobe agent of sorts whom I had hired for some strange reason, to help me buy all-new clothing. (There's another life-symbol buried in there if you can see it.) Together, we made our way to a shop and I began trying on this piece and that. A striped jacket with those pants. This shirt with that other tie. It was sort of fun, I admit.

When finished, I felt great. We left the store and proceeded to engage in a number of events, interacting with people and such, until a growing sense of discomfort began to eat at me. I wasn't sure exactly why, but I was not feeling entirely myself. Then, like a freight train, it hit me. As I looked down at myself, I realized I was wearing women's clothes.

"A dress! I'm wearing a dress!"

Not only that, but it was an entire woman's ensemble from the 1800's, puffy hairdo and all. I was mortified.

Strangely, nobody else seemed to notice or care. But I sure as hell did and I had to get out of those clothes as quickly as possible if not quicker. I searched around and found a side door that lead to the back room. Only as in a dream, the clothing that I had tried on in the store was somehow all there in the back, so I very quickly began rummaging through it, trying to find something, anything to wear. People kept wandering in to the back, interrupting me as I tried desperately to change my clothes. Finally, I was able to right the horrible wrong.

Now, dressed in a smart sports coat and tie, I walked confidently back out among all the people only to realize, I was also wearing a skirt and knee-high boots. Damn it! A tiny bit more masculine perhaps, I was still wearing women's clothes. (Aaaaaagh!) That's when I woke up.

Angry and confused, I spoke to the wardrobe consultant about it. "What in the world is happening?" I demanded. His response was not at all what I had hoped for. With an evil smirk, he offered, "Too bad…It's going to cost you a lot more now. Was $10…but now…more like $20,000." We had never discussed his fee and now, he had me over the proverbial barrel and was bilking me. I was incensed. There was nothing I could do. Standing there, dressed as a woman, I was completely screwed.

So, what does that all mean? That I'm a closet cross-dresser? I don't think so, not that there's anything wrong with that, I just don't really think that's the deeper meaning. (Although they were really nice boots.) No, it wasn't about clothing at all, women's or otherwise. It was about "change". The clothing in this dream was merely a symbol for my addiction to alcohol.

At the point in the dream when I suddenly realized it, seeing myself clearly for the first time, it made me horribly uncomfortable, despite the fact that nobody else seemed to mind. Regardless of anyone else's feelings, for the first time, it was my decision and I needed to change everything and immediately. But interestingly, even as I did attempt to change, costing me a small fortune, I still walked away, skirt and boots, wearing the remains of my alcohol. I may have wanted to change, but it didn't mean I didn't still have the lingering threat of my addiction.

Wow. Upon interpreting my own dream, the clarity I felt was like a light bulb in a dark room. My message to myself, loud and entertaining, was "be aware." Just because I had decided to quit drinking, doing quite well in my efforts by the way, it didn't mean the danger or the temptation to drink and the very real possibility that I would return to my old ways, was much closer than perhaps I realized. All I needed to do was look at myself a little closer to see, plain as day...I'm still wearing a damn dress.

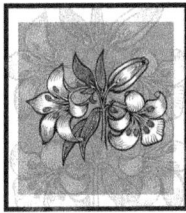

The Unimaginable Loss of
MARGARET B. KERCHEVAL

By the size of their gravestone, towering over all others in the Sacramento Historic Cemetery, a massive angel guarding from on top, it is evident that the Kerchevals made a little bit of money by coming out west. Traveling by wagon all the way from Missouri, like a million other hopeful gold-hungry treasure hunters, hitting the Sierra Nevada foothills in 1849, Reuben and Margaret Kercheval pressed on a bit further to find a vein of a different color. Fresh fruit.

While many people scoured the hills and rivers for their gold, the Kercheval clan focused on horticulture. Reuben's younger brother, Albert, came along for the journey and was instrumental in introducing the lady bug as a voracious warrior against notorious white scale insects that had dominated and destroyed previous attempts to grow fruit along the Sacramento River Delta and throughout Courtland where they planted their roots, so to speak.

Reuben prospered for close to thirty years after his arrival, but it was his wife Margaret who really brought it all home. After the death of her husband in 1881, she took to buying up great parcels of land along the river and increasing their orchards like a maniacal fruit lady.

Evidently, from the few records that remain, she did pretty well for herself and her children. Based on the size of the grave marker, either she had severe headstone envy, or was quite proud of her sizable accomplishments. And rightfully so.

The real story, however, the one that caught my eye, was that of the pain she must have endured along the way. Reading between the lines, it became evident that she was the mother of two small boys, Eddie and Choldsten, both of whom never made it past the age of six.

Coming all the way across the dangerous countryside, and building a veritable fruit empire, at the young age of 29, she gave birth to Edward H.S. Kercheval in 1863 only to lose him six short years later. How devastating and painful that must have been, I can't even begin to imagine.

In my wanderings throughout the massive cemetery, I came across countless gravestones in which lay the memories of small children. Some merely remembered as "Infant," not living long enough even to be named.

In my research, I found that there was a severe cholera epidemic in Sacramento sometime in the 1850's. Whether or not that was the reason for so many deaths or not, evidently many children struggled to survive those difficult days.

How exactly, little Eddy died remains a mystery. Very few knew the child and certainly nobody remembers him. His mother, however, no matter how strong of a pioneer woman she was, must have reeled at the loss.

But she was strong. Once again, eleven years later, in 1875, she gave birth to another son, Choldsen. Named after a distant relative from the old country, this new gift of life might have served to bring her up from the depths of her sorrow, only to toss it back in her face once again.

Choldsen, too, lived only six years. Like his brother, he was taken at such a young age and from a woman who had already experience the exact same pain only years before.

So, that's where I stop and take a moment to contemplate this sad story. Now only a name and a date etched into the granite, faded and worn with over a century of time, how does a person survive such trauma? All of her success, her ambitions and dreams, nothing could possibly compare to the intense loss of losing not one child, but two.

I currently have a six-year old as well as a five-year old boy. They are not babies with no names. They are not tiny infants who have not had the time to create an impact on me and lasting memories. They have become real people with stories of their own, sharing a life with me and my connection with them runs so deep, the very thought of losing them would kill me.

But this is exactly what happened to this woman, Margaret. People may happen upon her gravesite today and seeing the grandiose statue over her family's gravesite, imagine a rich story of great and lasting success. Very few would catch a glimpse of the real story of a cruel life in which her dreams were shattered by the continued loss of the children she loved so much. And yet, there it is, etched in stone, for anyone who takes the time and cares to see.

If there is any happiness remaining in her story, she had three other children to share her grief. James Louis was 10 years old when his little brother Eddie died. Howard Douglas was 9, and Hartley Henry, just 1 year old.

Standing upon this site, day after day, bearing the weight of my own failures and difficulties, I feel shallow, the weight of my burdens almost meaningless in the face of what this family endured. The perspective it provides me, yields no small sense of gratitude. My life, with all its ups and downs, the seeming overwhelming difficulties, the pain I have been dealt...I can manage.

In my searches, I was fortunate to stumble across the following long-forgotten poem written by Albert Kercheval. Clearly, it highlights the pain and suffering the family endured at the continually interfering hand of death.

Close the dreamless eyes that stare
With their vacant, rayless glare;
They are free from pain and care.

Lowly, gently o'er him bow,
Smooth the hair above his brow;
He is resting, sleeping now.

Resting from earth's ceaseless wear,
Resting from his weary care,
In the cold, white stillness there.

Breathe a prayer to Him to save,
While the funeral banners wave,
Bear him gently to the grave.

Softly, gently lay him low
Circling sadly, come and go,
In the spray of cypress throw.

In thy love, oh, God! We trust;
Here we lay thee with the just —
"Earth to earth, and dust to dust."

— Albert F. Kercheval

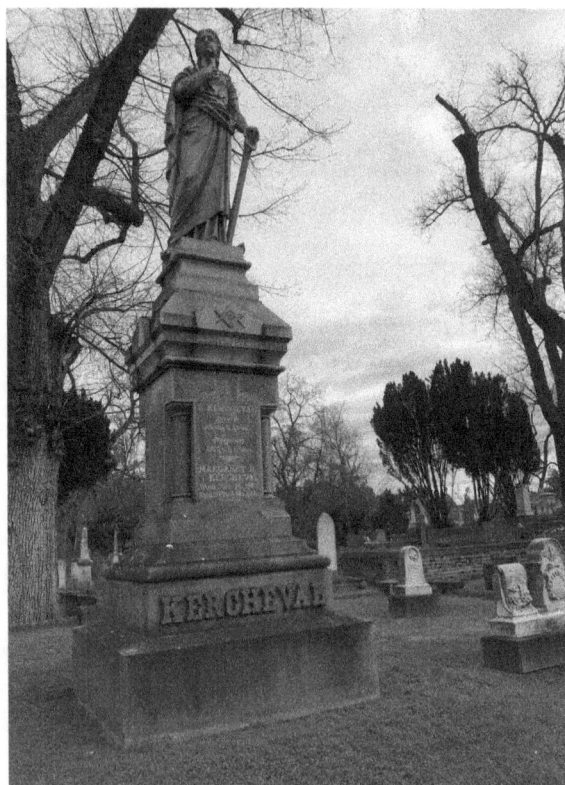

The Kercheval family plot guarded by an Angel.
Sacramento Historic Cemetery

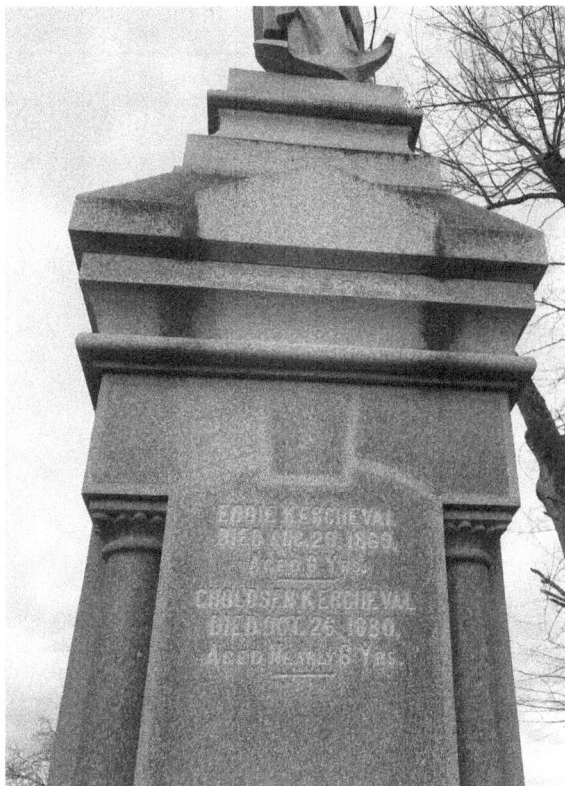

Kercheval grave marker – Insert of Eddie and Choldsen
Sacramento Historic Cemetery

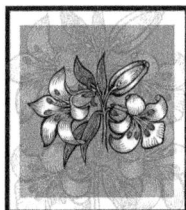

MY SISTER DIED TODAY

AUGUST 1, 2017

It was no surprise to anyone when Kathy died. A relief is more like it. That didn't make it any easier, though. My eldest sister, by five years, she was the first to go in a long line of Irish Catholic siblings. I know it's an inevitable part of life, inescapable, having the people you love die, but I had never experienced it yet, so close to home. We were always such a large, close-knit family. Six kids in all, and now…now there were only five.

I was staying on the California coast in a little town called Elk. It's become a second home to me and has been since my mid-twenties. Quiet, sleepy, rolling fog and crashing waves, it was a good place to sit and think, watch the ocean rolling in, rolling out again, and say good-bye to her.

I wasn't with her when she passed. My brother, John, told me over the phone, "There's no reason for you to come all this way. She won't know you're here." His words gave me the comfort and strength I needed to stay right where I was and talk to her as though she was sitting there right next to me.

Cancer, of course, is what took her down. Isn't that how most people go these days? It's a strange, ravaging disease that shows no mercy and takes no prisoners. It literally destroys a person, bit by bit, from the inside out. Kathy was an incredible person, but the cancer couldn't have cared less.

In her thirties, she had decided she'd had enough of the laborious, work-a-day world in which most of us waste our days. No, she decided she'd rather live her life with a paintbrush in her hand, and canvas after beautiful canvas, that's exactly what she did. In fact, that's all she did.

I always marveled at her courage and ability to "walk away from it all," so to speak, and live the simple life of a painter. I always wanted to do exactly that, but simply couldn't muster the courage. Of course, she never saw it that way. It wasn't courage that drove her, she just couldn't live her life any other way. And that's the biggest compliment I could ever pay anyone. Strangely, and outspoken about it, she was always so proud of me. Weird how that works.

My sister's death hit me in a very selfish way. It made me think about myself a lot, my own mortality, and that the window on my own life is quickly closing. Her dying like that, it means I don't have much time left either. And that's a little disturbing. Here I should be mourning for her, and all I can do is think about myself. That said, I know when to cut myself some slack. I know that's how it works. It's difficult, if not impossible, to witness the death of someone you love, try to draw some sort of meaning from it all, then apply it to yourself.

In this case, her willingness to go against the grain most of her life, pursuing the simplicity of her talents, painting for no other reason than that it made her happy, serves as an inspiration to me. Maybe I don't have to struggle so. Maybe I don't have to accomplish great things, building castles and empty empires. Maybe I just need to relax and enjoy the life that I've been given. The days that I have now. The few moments that remain.

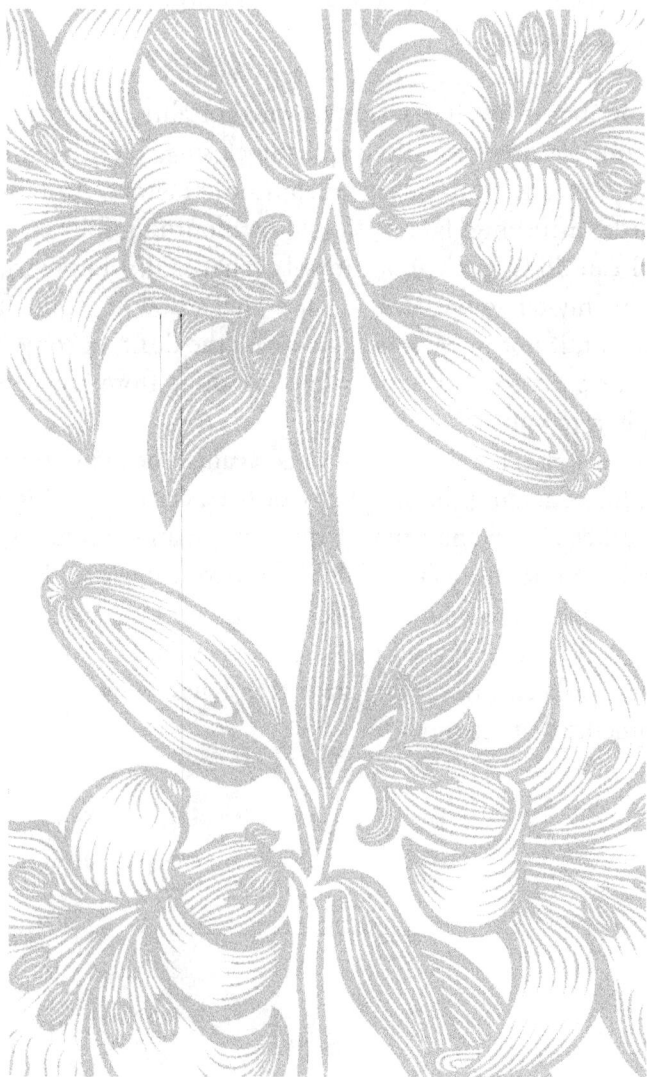

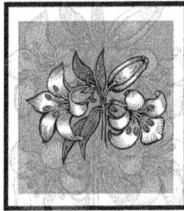

CLOSING DOWN
THE OL' GARAGE

———

DECEMBER 20, 2017

———

I live in a nice old neighborhood, just minutes from downtown. It reminds me of something snatched out of a Thomas Kinkade painting. Except for the long line of cars stacked bumper-to-bumper every evening, waiting to get home and eat dinner. Every day, however, sitting in that same line myself, I would pass by this little old, run-down, grease pit of an auto repair shop. I don't think it even had a name or a sign out front. With broken glass in several windows, hand-prints on the walls, and old rusty, forgotten auto parts piled off to the side, it was just a horrible little wart on the neighborhood. Leave it to me to come up with the stupid idea to save it.

But I couldn't stop thinking about it. Dreaming. Fantasizing how I could take this horrible excuse for a business, turn it around, and make my fortune. I would re-invent the greasy garage and soon, have another location just like it. Then another. And another. All up and down California and across the states, automotive repair would never be the same.

I partnered with an old friend, someone who had actual repair shop experience. I invested my money. Lots of it. And I invested my time and talents over eight long years building that place. Red Rocket Auto Tech. And it was gorgeous, I mean drop-dead gorgeous.

And lo and behold, everyone else seemed to love it, too. That long line of cars in my neighborhood, they started coming to my shop. They started telling their friends and family about it. The word got out, in auto repair, there was a new place, a special place, a non-greasy place you could trust. So, location number two seemed like a natural. That was the dream, after all, a string of these beautiful little places. I dug a little deeper, forked over more money, borrowed a chunk from a friendly bank who believed in us, burned a ton more time, and opened another location.

Fate, however, was not as kind to us this time. From the beginning, it felt like a dirty trick had been played on us. The new landlord threatened to take us to court just as we opened the doors, suing for back rent based on code issues, permits, and other city ordinances that took well over a year to resolve, ultimately preventing us from opening. All the while, money was leaking out of my pocket. Then, just when it couldn't seem to get any worse, my business partner and operations guy had a severe stroke. And it all started sliding downhill. Fast.

From January 1st through December 20th, we tried to hold it together. But without his daily involvement, the shop went to hell. The mechanics were thieves, stealing tools and equipment. The manager became lazy, preferring the interests of her Facebook page, unconcerned with whether or not customer's cars got fixed right the first time or not. She allowed the place to go to hell, engine parts, axles and grease lining the walls. In such a short amount of time, our reputation began to suffer and the customers who once loved us, who bragged about us…just stopped showing up. The balance sheet started tumbling down hill and what had taken eight long years to create, crashed almost overnight.

Everything except the whopping debt was gone, and with my partner struggling to put a simple sentence together, in throes of a deep and dark despair, I stood alone facing attorneys, and a once-friendly bank that had suddenly taken off its mask, revealing a hungry shark beneath. In addition, a long line of pissed-off vendors formed outside the door, demanding their money. The dream wasn't just over, it had suddenly become a full-blown nightmare.

If ever there was a good reason to drink, I now had a long and justifiable list of them. But strangely enough, I didn't turn to my standard vodka tonics to ease the pain. Not out of sheer willpower so much, or any particular strength I had managed on my own, but something else. Something had changed in me over the year in which, I knew, I just knew, booze was no longer the answer. Not for me. I could see clearly that, with all that had happened in the past year, the amount of pain I was enduring, alcohol could and would only serve to increase it on every level. Suddenly, I not only didn't want to drink, I was afraid of drinking.

How's that for a tiny bit of success? Out of the proverbial ashes, the phoenix, small and a bit insecure, rises, taking flight. It's encouraging, I'll tell you that much. And I needed every bit of encouragement I could get. The depressing thought did cross my mind, once or twice, hopefully not true, that it might be open phoenix season and there was a line of hunters with shotguns just waiting to blow me out of the sky. But so far…no sign of them.

I think the most interesting thing about this otherwise total disaster, the silver lining, is that I'm beginning to see what life without alcohol can look like. In the midst of some of life's worst scenarios, when dreams crumble, and life deals you a rotten hand, the absence of booze might just perhaps help me to go through it with more presence, more courage, and perhaps even a bit more grace, not drowning my woes, stumbling over myself, and making a bigger mess of it all along the way. This is not something I know. Rather, it is a feeling, a new sense of well-being that gives me strength.

If I dream a big dream and it doesn't come true, it's OK. I will survive. If I build a business and it fails, in the larger scope, it's really not that big of a deal. I can always build another one, or better, pick up a paint brush and paint something blue. Like the proverbial roller coaster ride, I can choose to white-knuckle the seat in front of me, scream in holy terror up and down and all around, and hang on for dear life until it finally stops. Or I can sit back, hold on, and enjoy the hell out of myself.

Just remember, keep your hands and feet inside the vehicle at all times.

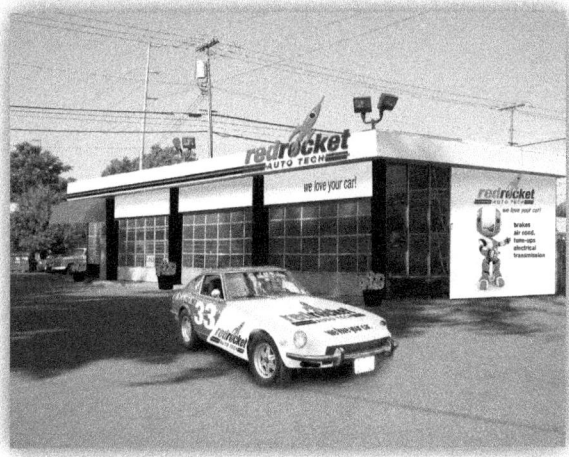

Red Rocket Auto Tech • 2009 - 2017
Sacramento, California

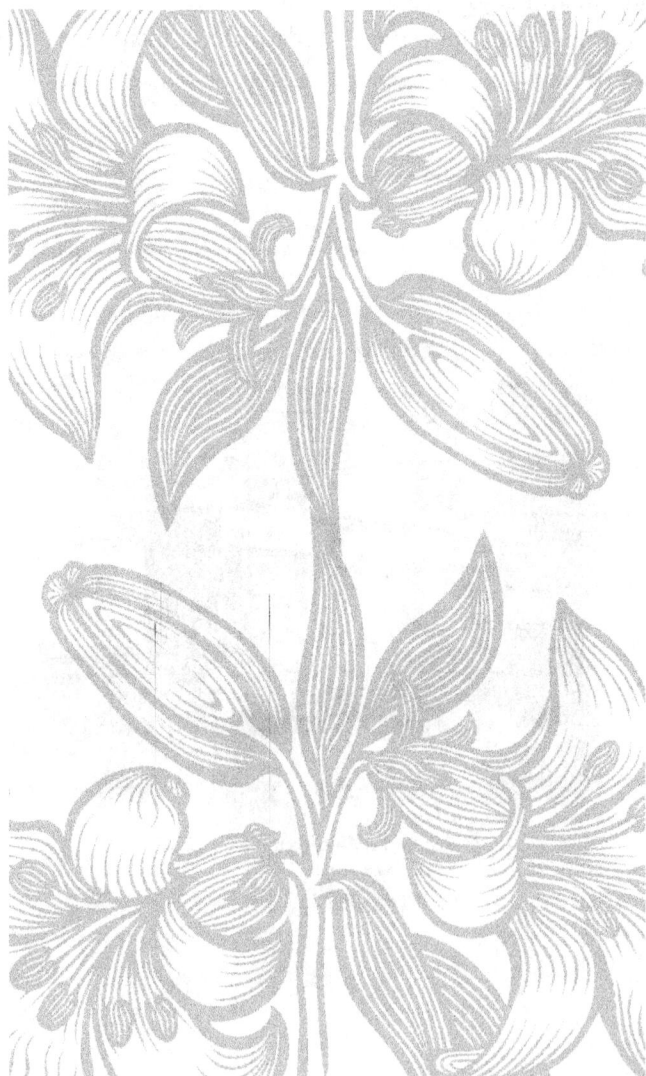

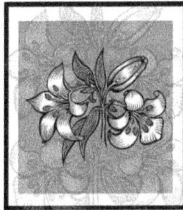

The Opium Habits of a Forgotten
CHINESE GENTLEMAN

I apologize for my lack of understanding Asian cultures.
To be perfectly frank, I cannot tell you if the person buried
beneath my feet was a man or a woman. By the markings on
the gravestone, I assume he or she was Chinese. With that in
mind, I will take a little creative liberty and guess at the story
around this person's life, including the theory that it was even a
man.

If you know anything about the Chinese during the time of
the old west, it is quite likely this person endured hardships the
likes of which most of us today will never know. Likely, one of

thousands of Chinese workers who helped lay the railroad from east to west, the honorable Mr. Chang, as I have named him, saw some pretty brutal days under the sun. But even prior to his unforgiving torture, laying mile after mile of steel tracks, he had to make his way to America first. Perhaps he would have been better off to stay in China drinking tea, but then again, perhaps not.

China was a country in dire trouble at that time. Not only had the Taiping Rebellion broken out, by far one of the bloodiest civil wars in history, but jolly old England, you see, had for hundreds of years prior been undermining the very moral fabric of a once beautiful land.

Fat, rich, and happy, England had done as much damage as it possibly could to India and decided China would make a rather splendid place indeed to wreak havoc and destroy next. Having completely decimated India, removing as much of her treasures as possible, shipping them back home, lining the pockets and castle walls of the bloated English aristocracy, they thought it would bring in substantial additional profits if they should turn to illegal drug smuggling.

Using the fertile land stolen from the peaceful people of India, they constructed endless farms and factories in the industrious effort to produce opium, ship it into the south China seas, then smuggle it up the myriad river channels into the very heart of China.

Outlawed by the Emperor for its devastating effect on his people, the English traders couldn't care less whether opium was legal or not. The fact that it was incredibly addictive and destroyed the lives of anyone who came near it was none of their concern either. There was a crapload of filthy lucre to be made and that was plenty reason enough.

With the amiable help of cutthroat pirates and other less scrupulous criminals, the English created a vast network of opium dealers and an illicit industry that made the English elite fatter than they could have imagined while stripping China of her dignity. Opium addiction became an epidemic, undermining the people as well as the government itself and coming very close to destroying the most honorable and ancient civilization from within.

In every sense of the word, these "respectable" entrepreneurial and industrious Englishmen, more specifically the East India Trading Company, or the Honorable Company as its Lords referred to it, became one of the first, possibly the largest drug cartel the world has ever known.

The French and Portuguese were not without sin, however, in this whole charade. But it was clearly the English who ruled the day and made out like bandits. (They were, in fact, literally bandits.) The East India Trading Company in particular, grew so wealthy off of their illegal opium trade, they eventually formed their own army and navy, one so large and feared by anyone who opposed them, that England relied upon them for protection. With their complete rape of India, this company became, in a sense, its own country.

So, our man, Mr. Chang… perhaps this is why he fled his beloved China. Maybe like the rest of us in America, he was simply trying to escape the English. For whatever reason, he found his way on board a ship and sailed for worlds unknown, never to see his home again, nor the people whom he loved. Whether he was a humble monk, a farmer, or a successful businessman, he packed his bag with whatever he could carry and risked his life to reach the shores of America, stepping foot on dry land, homeless, jobless, and within days of starvation.

But, lucky for Mr. Chang, the Chinese were welcome in America. Unlike the drunken Irish fools who stumbled off their boats, Chinese men could be counted on, working for pennies, and respectfully obedient, doing as they were told without much fuss. Stick a gazillion of these guys together, and you could create a miracle; as in the Transcontinental Railroad.

As he built the railroad for the next thousand years, coming to a grand finale in 1869, like many jobless Chinese laborers, he would have made his way to Sacramento to help build the Delta levees all up and down the Sacramento River. In a matter of time, these levees turned over 500,000 acres of useless swamp land into some of the richest farm land in California, making billionaires out of a few crafty farmers.

But like the railroad, the profits never graced Chinese pockets. Considered less than human, they just did all the work. Opium, however, as in their homeland, continued to bring substantial ease to their daily pains.

It is entirely possible Mr. Chang was an opium addict himself. Or, if he somehow had the strength and wisdom to avoid it, like the English, he may have used it to profit himself. Opium addiction didn't stay in China alone but traveled the seas right along with the hopelessly addicted immigrants, poisoning the new country as well. Opium dens popped up like Starbucks, one on every corner in every little town that the railroad passed through all across the fruited plains.

An 1860's excerpt from The Sacramento Union newspaper, while not condoning it use, likens opium to alcohol in its medicinal affects:

"There are many persons who cannot use alcoholic compounds, yet whose mode of life and occupations subject them to severe mental strain, rendering them liable to

frequent fits of nervous depression. To such as those, opium suggests itself as a ready means of relief..."

I love it. "Some people cannot use alcohol..." How unfortunate. But don't you worry... there's always opium to get you through the daily stresses of life. Many people have difficult jobs, you see, and it causes them no uncertain amount of depression. Ah, poor babies. Hey, I have an idea! You should smoke opium!

Who is to say whether opium is more addictive or dangerous than alcohol? They both are abused to treat the exact same symptoms. They are both used an escape from our lives, the stress, the boredom, the anxiety and depression. It's the same old story and, evidently, it's been taking place for centuries.

I do not really know anything about our friend Mr. Chang, whether he was an addict, a dealer, or a good church-going man...but if he was facing the struggles of life in those days, he no doubt had his hand in some pretty serious anesthetic solutions. How he died is anyone's guess. For the sake of my story, however, I suggest he smoked himself to death.

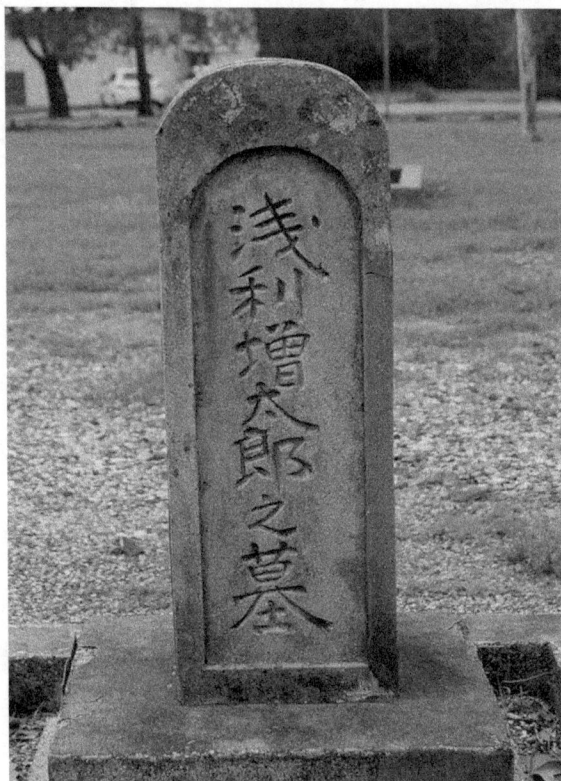

A Forgotten Chinese Immigrant – alias, Mr. Chang.
Sacramento Historic Cemetery

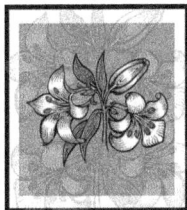

HAPPY FREAKIN' NEW YEAR

JANUARY 1, 2018

In a single year, 2017, likely the most difficult year of my entire life, I got arrested for driving under the influence, lost my driver's license, was sent to jail, watched my sister suffer and lose to cancer, had a business partner suffer a severe stroke, went bankrupt, and finally, in mid-December, closed the doors to my once-thriving, eight-year old business. My self-image crumbled, my family mourned, my friendship evaporated, insatiable banks and attorneys chewed on my ankles, and any entrepreneurial dreams I ever dared have, or the hope of a solid retirement, suddenly blew away in the wind.

And somehow, I was able to endure all of this...without a drink in my hand. I'm not sure how, but in some miraculous way, I went through some of the biggest fires and all at the same time, without turning to booze.

Funny, in the past, any one of those situations would have been the perfect excuse to grab a drink and ease the pain. Cocktails with a friend would actually have been quite the prescription for relief. I mean, the stuff works, after all. The truth, now becoming more apparent every day, is that, while it does ease the pain, like any anesthetic, it only masks what is truly there. Yes, I'd heard that analogy many times before, but it was meaningless, falling on deaf ears. Yeah, I'm masking the damn pain, so what?

But honestly, that is coming from a personal perspective that pain is a bad thing. What if it isn't? What if pain, as uncomfortable and much as it hurts, were a means to help us, change us, guide and direct us...meant for our ultimate good? Then maybe masking it is self-destructive after all. Maybe not feeling the pains of life is a way of holding me back. The more and more I ease my own pain and suffering, a drink or two at a time, the more I stay right where I am, never growing as a person, never realizing the new joys and opportunities that might be waiting for me, right around the corner. I didn't see it clearly then. I was too numb.

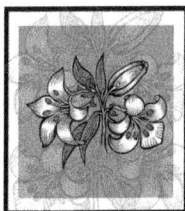

ATTACHED TO OUTCOMES

The disaster I faced in the ultimate closure of my auto repair shop, *Red Rocket*, was increasingly difficult and more painful than it needed to be, not because of the financial difficulties I faced, rather, the emotional attachments I had, specifically the ways in which it "was supposed" to turn out.

Well of course I did! A chain of thriving auto centers, millions of dollars, and a fat, little retirement nest egg... that was the vision, my dream, my secret safety net in case nothing else panned out. Damn right I was emotionally attached.

And while nobody in their right mind would question such an attachment, it's perfectly normal after all, I can see clearly now how it became the root of added pain to the whole experience of losing my shop. And if that's true, how often does this same sort of attachment in other areas and efforts, rear its disappointed head in my life?

The answer…daily.

All day long, every single day of every month, year after year after year.

For many years now, I have become increasingly familiar with the Buddhist teachings of "attachment," or letting go of predetermined outcomes. It's a very interesting, freeing way of approaching our lives. They talk about the natural human tendency for desire, wanting something, or reaching for something as I did in creating my automotive empire, but then stepping back and consciously detaching from its outcome. That sounds ridiculously impossible, doesn't it? I mean, it's not really human to be able to do such a thing. Wouldn't that make you into some sort of emotionless robot?

In practice, not really. In fact, it's just the opposite in that it frees up your emotions when they are not sunk so deep in holding onto something, especially when that something is slipping away; a business, a career, a marriage, even a family member. When we have it all figured out, exactly how it is supposed to turn out, and then it doesn't…emotionally, we crash. We become filled with anger, bitterness, resentment. We become indignant and closed off.

And honestly, detaching so to speak, isn't that exactly what we do when we drink to ease the pain? Not from our intended outcomes, but definitely from the pain of loss and suffering. We are, in every sense, attempting to escape it, get rid of it, hide from it. When in reality, if we were somehow able to detach ourselves from the ways in which things are "supposed to be" and ultimately are not, then the pain subsides naturally all by itself.

Pain and suffering, according to a Buddhist perspective, are a direct result from being attached to a million different things in our lives. Adding to that thought, pain and suffering are a few of the main reasons most drinking problems arise. We try to snuff out the flames in any way we can, as quickly as we can.

So, if drinking our problems away is no longer an option, as in my case, the alternative is either to suck it up like a big boy, face the pain head-on and just grit my teeth through it. Or perhaps I could learn to chill out a bit, let go of what I so desperately want and think I need, and simply allow what is…to be what it is.

Stupid Monkey

This reminds me of the story of the Hunter and the Monkey. By their very nature, monkeys are very quick on their feet, making them extremely difficult to catch. The wise hunter, however, is well aware of their greedy nature and one-track-mind when it comes to food and uses this insight against them. If a monkey sees something it wants, that very prize can quickly become its ultimate undoing.

Using a simple container, fixed by a chain or rope, with an opening large enough for the monkey to insert its hand, but small enough to prevent removal of the same hand when it is clenched, a fist, as holding on to something… then placing a piece of desirable food at the bottom of the container, the monkey then, in every sense, reaches in and traps itself.

Free to escape at any moment simply by letting go of the highly desirable morsel, it chooses instead to hold on for dear life, paralyzing itself, its clenched fist the only thing keeping it from freedom.

Seeing it through this lens, we are all just a bunch of monkeys. I sure as hell am. I've been grabbing at yummy chunks of food my whole life, holding on as tight as I could, demanding that life turn out a certain way and produce specified results, never realizing the power available to me, the freedom, if I would just have the insight, the wisdom, and the courage... to let go.

"Ah, bullshit," you say. "Detachment from outcomes is nothing more than a gooey, new age, cop-out. Like all religious mumbo jumbo, it's just a crutch for weak people to lean on." And maybe you're right. But for so many years, my old buddy vodka was a pretty dependable crutch as well. Only that crutch snapped and left me lying on a jail cell floor.

A crutch is not a bad thing. It sounds like it should be, after all nobody wants to walk around limping on a stupid crutch. The truth, however, it is an amazingly simple and effective tool created to help us walk when we are unable. And that's precisely the point. In life, so many times, the pain and suffering we face immobilizes us to the point that we cannot take another simple step forward. We need that damn crutch. As a result, so many, like me, turn to the most immediate and very effective form of pain killer we can find; booze. It works, and it works so well.

But the effects are temporary. They don't last. And as all us die-hard drinkers know, too well, a good binge always brings a lot more problems to the party. So then, is the concept of letting go, or detachment from specified outcomes, a simple disguise for some Buddhist philosophical crutch? Maybe. Call it what you want. But, like alcohol, it's pretty effective, too. Only its effects are long term and lasting. Best of all, there's no nasty hangover the next morning and the taste of a dead dog in your mouth.

In short, there's nothing wrong or unhealthy with desire. We all want things and want them badly. That's human. But we get all caught up in exactly how that desire is supposed to unfold and happen for us, and when it doesn't, we throw our tantrums, we cry out that life is so unfair, we clench our proverbial fist, kick and scream like a monkey, and wallow in our container of self-induced pain.

But then, how are we supposed to accomplish anything? Great question.

The monkey, in desperately grabbing at the food in the bottom of the container, inevitably traps itself, thereby becoming somebody else's pet, or worse, dinner. So, what's the alternative? Walk away and pretend the food doesn't exist or that he really had no interest in it to begin with? Absolutely not.

If the monkey is willing to let go, it has all the time in the world to sit there, examine the situation, the container, its contents, and just possibly, the option of another approach. He could simply tip the container over on end, dumping the food out. He could smash the container with a rock, exposing it. He could even reach in and take smaller pieces, with a little patience, removing them bit by bit. Given the time he has each day to sit in the sun and play, a wise monkey might invent a thousand different creative ways to get at that food. But no, he already has the answer, or so he thinks, and he refuses to let go.

———————————

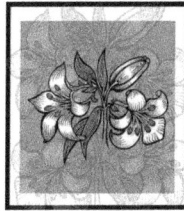

HAPPY BIRTHDAY, DAD

———

FEBRUARY 4, 2018

———

SuperBowl Sunday, my Dad came to town, celebrating his 90th birthday. Rather, we celebrated it, his children, because he wasn't all that happy about it. Truth is, he has never been all that happy about anything. My dad is a dark figure in my life, a shadow, strange and distant. I know he loved me, but it was difficult for him to show it. We were never close, he and I.

During the football game, it became increasingly apparent to me and the rest of my family that he had slipped rapidly into his old age, dementia revealing its ugly face. It wasn't until after I returned home that my sister, Terry, confided in me that my own father had not known who I was. We had joked together, shared a laugh or two. I had even given him a hug before leaving and, thinking about it now, likely all that crossed his mind was, "Why is this strange man with a beard hugging me?"

He had chosen a hard life, my Dad. And life had been hard on him in return. What I do know about him, and it's not much, is that he started out as a rough and tumble kid up in Billings, Montana. Charles Flanagan, Jr.

His mother had died giving birth to his younger brother, Joey, and as a result, their family had been torn apart from the beginning. His father became a hopeless alcoholic, eventually killing him, and that was probably reason enough for my Dad to enlist in the US Air Force before he was even eighteen. Like many of that era, he lied about his age and the armed forces looked the other way. He was just another soldier; a body to be shot at.

Before he was twenty years old, he was a full-blown fighter pilot, flying massive jets and dropping bombs, obliterating one Korean village after the other, killing hundreds, if not thousands of people with no names. I can only imagine what that would do to a man, young or old. But he was still just a kid. A once innocent child who never knew his mother, lost his father to a bottle, then strapped in a giant flying bomb, and ordered to keep his finger on the red button, killing as many people as he possibly could.

That's got to leave a mark.

After the SuperBowl party, gathering together with my brother and sister, discussing the inevitable need to move him up closer to us, find a nice retirement community, it was shared that my Dad had a military pension coming to him, one that he had never touched. As it turns out, he had been given an honorable discharge on the basis of certain psychological trauma incurred during the course of the two wars in which he served. It was then pointed out that it wasn't just the constant bombing, or the stress of flying and fighting in the air that snapped a nerve, it was his final military assignment that broke the camel's back.

What finally drove my father over the edge was repeatedly knocking on a stranger's door; opened by the hopeful wife of a soldier coming home to his family, relaying the same message over and over, that her husband had been killed in battle. My Dad's job, completely unbeknownst to me and hearing it for the first time, was to tell countless families that their beloved husband and father would not be coming home again.

This, evidently, was more than he could handle, and he finally snapped. The Air Force kindly set him out on the doorstep, a small pension in his pocket and pat on the head. But, too proud, too bitter, or too broken…he never even accepted it. Not a single penny. He also never spoke a word about any of it. Not to his family anyway.

Often, based on our curiosity and genuine interest, when pressed for details he would flare up, go into a sudden rage, and change the subject. We learned early on, we were not allowed to talk about his past, certainly not about war. As a result, war occupying most of my Dad's life up to that point, we knew almost nothing about him. He became this strange, dark, angry monster who was to be avoided whenever possible.

Hitting him square in the forehead with a frying pan, nearly killing him, my mother divorced him when I was fifteen. It happened, so it seemed, in the course of a single afternoon. She smacked him with the greasy skillet, he packed his bags, tossed what he had in the back of his car, and headed down the driveway. And that was it. He drove as far as he could before shutting off the engine, finally, somewhere back under the big skies in the heart of Montana.

After that, for the next forty years, I saw him once, maybe twice each year. A phone call at Christmas. A nice card on my birthday. That became the extent of my relationship with my father. No wonder he didn't recognize me at the stupid SuperBowl game. He never knew me to begin with.

Sadder still, I never knew him either.

I share this story, however, not to wallow in my own self-pity, quite the contrary. It serves, selfishly, like my sister's death, as a reflection on my own life, providing insights and a new perspective. Like so many of us, I get all caught up in the pain and difficulties of my daily world, narrow-mindedly seeing myself as the center of the universe. I face endless and towering mountains, unfair and unplanned, and I feel sorry for myself. Stepping back, then, seeing my father's life, the perils, pain and suffering he endured, I am suddenly ashamed. My life is beautiful in comparison, and much to his credit.

When my father was twenty years old, he was flying a death machine, fighting for his life in wars, the innocent pawn of some war-monger General, listening to the sounds of bombs exploding beneath him, ending the lives of countless people. Me…when I was twenty years old, I was spending my days down on the American River, basking in the warmth of the California sun, smoking pot and flirting with girls in bikinis, listening to the sounds of Led Zeppelin, wondering where the party was that night. What right do I have, to ever get depressed about how difficult my life has been or will be? What do I know about pain? What losses have I ever endured that come even remotely close to those of my father? It shames me.

But in the same breath, it now enlightens me, encourages me, strengthens me, and reminds me…how fortunate I really am. It lightens my load. Eases any burden. I have been given an incredible life. With this perspective, I am nothing if not extremely fortunate. And the plain truth is, I owe a great deal of this to my father. He paid a heavy price for me. I have no room to complain about anything. Ever.

Therein, lies the moral to this story. There's always a new perspective we can bring to bear. When faced with the never-ending trials and tribulations that are life itself, we can choose to become self-centered, washing ourselves in self-pity, accept the bitterness that creeps in, and grow angry at the world.

And when it comes to alcohol, in my case and that of many others, it serves then to be the perfect antidote. Booze is a fantastic cure. It makes the symptoms of this selfish pain subside, even if for a moment. But with a broader perspective, and thoughts of gratitude, rather than a bad attitude, in the absence of alcohol this same pain can bring a new sense of life, growth, and appreciation for all that we have, and the strength to wake up and face anything that might come our way.

For the record, whether he ever reads these words, close relationship or not... I owe a great deal to my father.

Thank you, Dad.

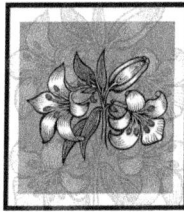

Stress, Anxiety, and Other
DEPRESSING DOLDRUMS

You could add boredom to the list, along with a number of other emotional responses to life that cause people to turn to booze for relief, but stress, anxiety, and depression are likely at the very top. I know they were for me.

The daily stress I have lived with over the last several decades is substantial. Perhaps not more so than any other human on the planet, but I have had a difficult time coping with raising six children, building a handful of companies, dealing with employees, attorneys, accountants, and non-stop government bullshit, family crisis after family crisis, a vindictive money-hungry ex-wife…the list is as endless as it is uninteresting and irrelevant to you. My point is that life has been a bumpy ride for me, and I learned to let the pressure out of the kettle by drinking.

It's quietly seductive because it appears to work so well. Any edge simply dissolves upon that first sip. A couple cocktails into the afternoon and your worries all but disappear. Even the good old Bible tells us, *"Take a little wine for your many ailments…"* I always loved that one. It *"covered a multitude of sins"* and gave me free license to drink as I saw it.

Strangely enough, however, after a time, the more I drank to relieve those pressures, the alcohol began to add to them. Take depression for example, I never stopped to think about the fact that alcohol by its very nature is a clinical depressant. I had no idea (or concern) what that even meant. For me, it meant I often carried around a little dark cloud of personal gloom over my head. After seeing me drag my feet around the house and sighing deeply over and over, my wife would often ask me what was wrong. Often, there was really nothing in particular upsetting happening, no crisis, just living in the dumps.

It wasn't until a few months after I quit drinking, when my system began to clear, that I noticed a strange sense of lightness begin to take shape, like the fog beginning to lift. It wasn't miraculous, but it was noticeable. And nothing else in my life had changed for the better to quantify it, in fact, quite the opposite what with all the court and legal issues, fines and jail time I was facing. Life was not pretty whatsoever and yet, somehow, I began feeling less depressed. Go figure.

I drank to escape depression and became increasingly depressed as a result. Pretty stupid prescription. So, a dose of reality then. How the hell are we supposed to deal with the intense pressures of adult life, self-induced or otherwise, if we can't drink them away? If we don't relieve the mounting pressures, something's going to blow somewhere.

The horrible lie with booze is that it keeps you from finding those answers. The truth is, there are many ways to relieve emotional pressures, but under the cloak of alcohol, you'll likely never find them. It teaches us how to solve our issues but in a very thin, addictive, and increasingly ineffective manner.

Actually, feeling the cold, hard pain of life in and of itself is not a bad place to start. Reality, as much of a bitch as it can be, is a real eye-opener and will teach us, if we let it, which direction we should turn. Like the proverbial "hand over the burner" if we couldn't feel the pain of the hot stove, we'd simply keep our hand in the flame and burn to death. It's that first sign of searing pain that causes us to yank our hand back. In that sense, pain is a fantastic gift and a very effective deterrent.

Another effective and far more lasting approach to facing the daily stresses of being alive, is awareness of the stress itself. Simple clarity as to how I am feeling. Perhaps, not even why I am feeling stressed, even though that will provide even more clarity, but just knowing that I am stressed can help me to step back and look at it. Admit it to myself. This alone lets off a little steam. If I know I'm stressed, then maybe I can spend a few moments and figure out the source of it, contemplate it, and realize it's not so bad after all.

Too often, stress will sneak in the back door and not announce itself, creeping up behind and wrapping itself around us without our even being aware of it. We become ignorantly tied up in a little knot, chewing our fingernails and pulling out our hair and we have no bloody reason why. We feel the stress, but never identify it. All we want is the pain to go away. Nothing a good stiff drink won't solve. And of course, temporarily, it does just that. The edge melts quickly away and we never even took the opportunity to see that we were stressed. Or why. With booze, we fix the problem before we ever even know we have one. There's a term for that. I call it self-induced blindness.

There are times, however, when it is painfully obvious that we are so damn stressed out and we even know exactly why. "I have no money, I've missed three payments, and the bank is threatening to repossess my pants! Yeah, I'm stressed out of my freaking head and there is no relief in sight! None! Now give me a damn drink!"

That's the kind of real stress that produces a deeper anxiety. Like fear and torment, the anxiety begins to eat away at you, telling you there are no answers available. Your world is coming to an end. There is no solution. No hope. You might as well just throw in the towel. "But before you do that," your little friendly addiction whispers, "you may consider going and grabbing a cocktail or two. That's always a good idea, right? Of course, it is. Besides, you've been working so hard and life is so damn unfair, if you don't deserve a good shot down the ol' gullet, nobody does." And so, two best friends, just you and your addiction, head off to the nearest bar for a spoonful of medicine.

One day leads to the next, the stress and anxiety never cease, but the bar tab keeps growing. And your drinking habits steadily increase, year after year after year, until one day, you sit up and entertain what so many well-meaning people have been saying behind your back and your best drinking buddies will never tell you… "Dude, you've got a problem."

But of course, sly as it is, that old voice is the first to talk you out of such nonsense. "Even if you do have a drinking problem," it promises, "surely it isn't a bad one. You could quit drinking any time you wanted to… just not now. Maybe you can take a booze break, ease off in a few weeks, but for now, it's way too stressful. You need a drink…" Sounds logical. Good advice. You buy into it and, boom, you're off to the races one more time.

The key to dealing with severe anxiety is to face it head on. Step naked through the fire. In some recent adventures dealing with multiple hungry attorneys, all gnawing at me, threatening impending lawsuits, escalating legal fees and torturing my dog just for fun, I was faced with some real anxiety issues. But over the course of the last year, not turning to alcohol for relief, I have been learning to deal with the pain in an all new way, something my addiction never allowed me to experience. It's incredibly hard, but has produced a growing sense of calm, almost faith if you can believe in such a thing, that there is light at the end of the tunnel. Pressing through the pain, reaching for that little light, has made me stronger, ever so slightly.

I meditate now. (Freaky, I know.) But so many people are into it these days, it's not like I've gone rogue and become a flipped-out hippie or something. (I am a flipped-out hippie by the way.) Plus, it actually works. Not as immediately as whiskey or vodka, true, but it does have a controlled, soothing effect. It has a way of providing clarity around a number of different areas of my life, and clarity, well that has become my favorite subject. Plus, there's no nasty side effects like getting tossed in the slammer for it. Like drinking, I don't necessarily recommend it while driving, but as a more holistic and longer-lasting solution, practiced in the privacy of your own home, it's a fairly decent one.

———————

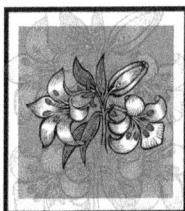

Looking in the Mirror
PRECIOUS SELF IDENTITY

When I began my career in advertising, I was just a kid, twenty-five years old, had never finished college, had no degree (which everyone told me was the most important thing in the world), and two children to feed. To be blunt, I was scared to death.

But somehow, I was able to put a few puzzle pieces together, one here, another there, and build both a business and a career. As it turns out, I was good at both. I taught myself, buying book after book, learning my trade and applying what turned out to be my own unique brand of creativity. Things started looking good. I won awards and lots of them and my reputation began to spread. It felt good.

My identity began to form around all this. The more my business grew, the more awards and acclaim I received, including *Advertising Executive of the Year*, the better I felt about myself. No college degree, true, but just look what I had accomplished. And while a positive self-image is important, an identity is something altogether different and not really who we are deep inside. That took a whole lot longer to find. In fact, I'm still digging.

In an earlier chapter, I revealed the story of Kevin Ramos and how, after losing his legs, and almost losing his life, like a rose in spring, he somehow managed to blossom, becoming a rare and inspiring example of a man in touch with a far deeper identity than simply a man with legs who could do things as well or better than other men with legs. No, Kevin was made of something far different, and somehow, perhaps through his pain and suffering, was able to find and hold onto something more real. Something of greater value.

I wish I could say the same thing about John Hutchinson, my friend and partner in my automotive business. When he suffered his stroke, it not only took him out of the game physically, it destroyed him emotionally as well.

John was, for all intents, a proud man. He was an unstoppable doer, self-made, entrepreneurial dynamo. Not much could stop him. He was a veritable bulldozer of a man. When going out to dinner, he would often make reservations using the name, Senator Hutchinson, something I always found down right hilarious. That was just the way John moved through life.

Unfortunately, he took it a bit more seriously than I realized. His identity and self-worth were very tied to all of this, so much so, that when the rug was yanked out from underneath him, suffering that debilitating stroke, he crashed, fell down, and refused to get back up. Unlike Kevin Ramos, John went the opposite direction, becoming darker and colder, cutting off the world and his friends. He became increasingly bitter. He hated the entire world and himself and wore it on his sleeve like a bloody bandage.

Trust me, John is not a bad person. I've known him for over thirty years. He is a good man. But, his self-identity was based on something unreal and paper thin so that, when it was taken from him, he lost everything. My genuine hope for John, is that he will continue this journey, not give up, and find something deeper within himself, come out the other side and, like Kevin, a better, stronger person because of it all.

Not to point fingers at John, I think much of the same was true of me. When I came to the realization that I had to quit drinking, my identity came into question. How in the world could I live a life without a drink in my hand? I'm Irish Catholic for crying out loud! I'm an advertising executive! That combination says booze no matter how you spell it. All my social and business relationships revolved around cocktails. Drinking was a way of life and I closely identified with it. To push that aside felt as if I was pushing a part of my soul aside.

But, seeing clearly now, that is preposterous. Drinking is not who I am. That's one of the reasons I dislike the title "alcoholic" because it tends to classify and identify a person, when in actuality, it does neither. Yes, I am a person who has a history of increasing problems revolving around alcohol, even an addiction to it, but in no sense of the word does it have anything to do with who I am.

Likewise, I am not defined by my Irish heritage, nor my Catholic upbringing, nor my career as an ad man. None of those are who I am. If I can learn to disassociate my identity with these very meaningful aspects of my life, then perhaps I can continue along those lines, ridding myself of all the meaningless layers that do not really identify me. Then, if the worst should happen, if the rug is yanked from beneath my feet, I will still be me. Only death can take that away, and even that's debatable.

———

For the sheltered Millenials in the room, in the film *On the Waterfront*, actor Marlon Brando, in a moment of raw clarity, tells his brother his simple truth and how he really feels about himself. *"You don't understand... I coulda had class. I coulda been a contenda. I coulda been somebody instead of a bum, which is what I am. Let's face it."*

———

You can see the restrained pain in Brando's face. But interestingly, you can also see him, in realizing his own truth, begin to let it go. He is not angry at his brother, the one "responsible" for his failure. He is broken, yes, but coming to grips with it, beginning to heal. The stardom he so desired as a professional boxer, and rightfully should have seen, was taken from him by somebody else. In this case, his own brother.

The pain he feels, is the pain we all feel when life is so unfair to us and doesn't give us what we think we deserve.

We work so hard. We struggle so much. We dream so big. Then life…it kicks us right smack in the teeth and laughs at us for daring to be so foolish. How the hell are we supposed to feel? Giddy? Are we supposed to get up and do a little jig when the roof falls in on our house? It hurts.

So, allow me to change the channel. Let's try a different approach. Let's say you are Brando and all you ever wanted was to be a boxer. But not just any boxer…the best boxer the world has ever known. Boxing is the single most important love of your life. And, for one reason or another, fair or unfair, you got the shaft. Your one big dream and life just spits in your face.

Then, what if a wise old soothsayer was to come along and tell you (Brando), "I realize this appears to be the end of the world and is more painful than you can bear. But because you have failed as a boxer," the old sage continues, "you will now travel a different road than the one you were on. You will meet a beautiful woman on that road, fall in love like you can't imagine, get married and father an incredible baby boy. You will love that boy, and cherish a lifetime of moments with him, raising him, coaching him and teaching him how to box as you once did."

Then, the prophet quietly provides one last, key insight that sets the stage for a whole new way of seeing. "Because of you," he declares, "and because of your failure, this young boy will grow to become the greatest boxer the world has ever known. The entire world will know his name. And you…his coach, father, and lifelong best friend."

Now, given the choice, his own fleeting stardom or that of his unknown, currently unplanned, yet-to-be-born son…how do you suppose Brando might respond? And what about that overwhelming pain he was wallowing in, what would happen to it? If Brando, in his moment of greatest suffering would allow himself to let go, just a little, and entertain the slim prospect that there just might be another outcome to what he had already so carefully planned… his pain would dissolve like honey in hot tea, gentle, soothing and sweet to the taste.

Nice tidy Hollywood ending, I know. But for those who prefer a strong dose of the real world, that's not always how it works. We all don't get to experience the happy ending.

Sometimes, we never get to see the whole picture and our lives, are just plain difficult, beginning to end. The resulting pain is, more often than not, still tied to our expected outcomes and our fist-shaking challenge to life that it should treat us fairly. As if it owes us something. We want, we demand, that life be a merry-go-round, filled with the delightful sounds of juke box music, decorated with pretty balloons, going 'round and 'round, laughing all the way. When suddenly, one of the gears on the carousel snaps and our horse throws us off, hitting the pavement with our forehead. We then struggle to get up, wipe the blood from our face and curse the wretched amusement park for ever tempting us with such a ludicrous and dangerous contraption.

Well, that's ridiculous and selfish. Fair or unfair, nobody ever claimed a merry-go-round was perfectly safe. Nobody intentionally destroyed our dreams. Somebody simply forgot to lube it properly and a gear broke, as gears often do. We can get angry, indignant, maybe even attempt to sue the amusement park for a million dollars, but in the end, it doesn't change the truth. We just happened to be on the wrong pony at the wrong time.

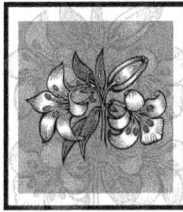

Finances and Familiar Fiascos
LIFE'S LITTLE HURDLES

Money sure is a funny thing. It's more than precious to us and we closely identify with "our" money. You can call me names, kick me in the shins, or throw rocks at me, but screw around with my money and I will go bananas on you. So much of our identity and self-worth is tied up in something so fleeting, and candidly, so unreal, that it demands a little of our attention here as we look at becoming "disconnected" with the outcomes in our life.

Why do we care so much about how much we make each year, or how fat our bank account has grown, or not grown, as the case may be? We consider ourselves successful to a certain self-imposed degree based on how much money we have acquired. Almost more than anything else, we allow it to determine who we are. Our identity and personal net worth become intertwined and wrapped up in financial net worth.

Over this last year, as my entrepreneurial efforts in the auto business crumbled before my eyes, I watched in horror as eight years of hard work went up in flames. But it was the aftershock, after it was all gone, when I still was facing angry creditors, banks, and lawyers and having to reach deep into my pockets to make them go away and leave me alone, tapping the hard-earned cash I had saved for years. They were stealing my money. Or that's how it felt.

In every sense of the word, I was feeling abused, taken advantage of, and bilked of what was rightfully mine. They, on the other hand, saw it exactly the opposite. It was "their" money. The very thought of it, even now, makes my stomach turn. So why is that? Why do I really care who gets what in the end?

Looking back at all those thousands upon thousands of gravestones in the old cemetery, who remembers who made how much and who owed what to whom? It's all gone now. Nobody cares. Even the richest of the rich are still lying six feet below the dirt. None of them are any richer or better off than anyone else lying next to them, once rich, or stone cold flat broke.

We know it doesn't matter, and yet, we allow money to dictate our emotions, how we see and value ourselves, and whether or not we are happy. It's total unadulterated bullshit.

Sometime in my forties, I had a sudden epiphany, a realization that as much as I had worried about my finances over the decades, I really never lacked for anything. There was always enough money to eat and play and enjoy myself. I even paid my bills for the most part. Outside of being filthy rich and doing whatever I please whenever I pleased, money seemed to be adequate. In that realization, something clicked in me, a small internal voice, that assured me, I was going to be OK.

That insight slowly turned into a life philosophy, a humorous joke at first, but then began to solidify into a perspective that, when faced with difficult financial situations, I'd say to myself… "Oh, well. I will just need to make some more money to cover it." It sounds a bit weird, perhaps, but I've ingrained it into my mindset to the point, I actually believe it now.

I would like to tell you that money does not matter to me anymore. And while that is where I would like to be, emotionally, it's not true. My identity and my self-worth still have far too many green tentacles wrapped around my heart. But, if awareness means anything, at least I can see it. At least I am conscious of my desire to be free of a concern for money and minimize the emotional states into which it often pulls me. Perhaps, that is a step or two in the right direction.

———————

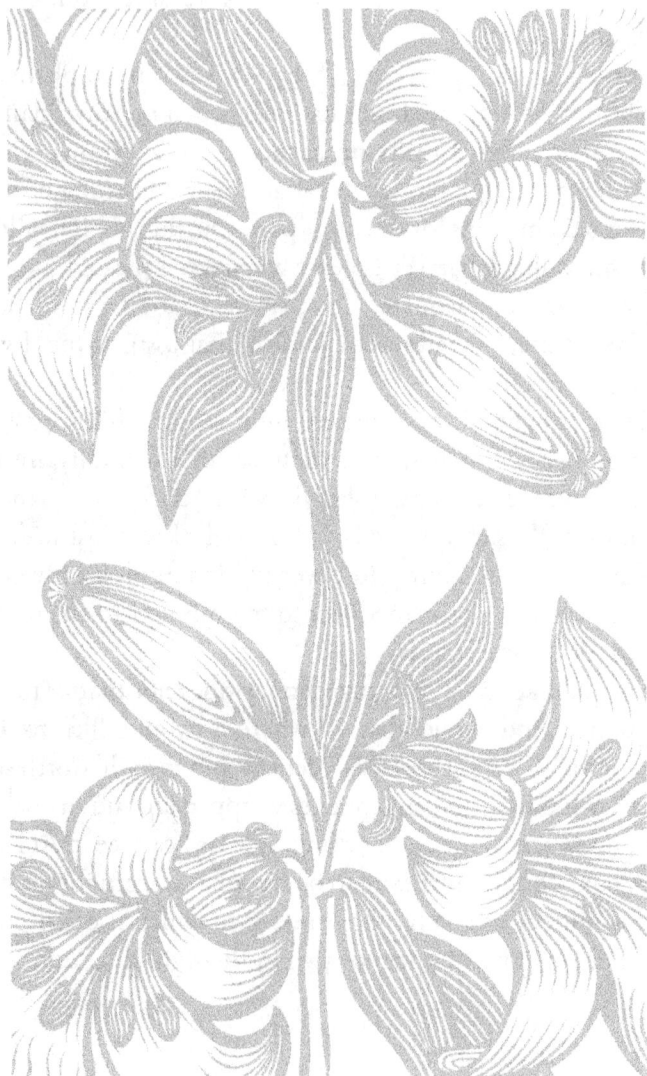

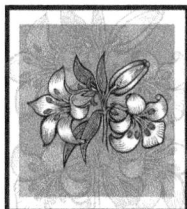

The Ancient Art of
DRINKING TOO MUCH

*What's the difference between an Irish wedding
and an Irish funeral?*

(One less drunk.)

As I mentioned, growing up in an Irish Catholic family.
Alcohol was everywhere. It was a part of life. A basic food
group. Everybody drank and lots of it. But unlike many
people, I never learned how to drink responsibly, regardless
of what all the friendly advertisers recommend. I was not
endowed with a filter or a recognizable limit that notified
me when I'd had too much to drink. Others could clearly
see it, but not me. I just simply kept on drinking until either

the booze was all gone, or I simply passed out. And it's been that way since I was roughly fourteen years old.

I have always been amazed by my wife, Karin, in her incredible ability to pour herself a single glass of wine, then only drink half of it. Who does that? How do you do that? Me…I would polish a bottle off by myself and go to the cellar for another.

Speaking of cellars, I tried for the longest time to maintain a robust wine cellar in my basement. It was the perfect place for it, plenty of room, the perfect temperature, with one small exception - I couldn't keep it stocked. I drank everything.

I think if I had been taught how to drink, perhaps I would not have faced so many problems around alcohol. But as it was, I had to teach myself and did a pretty piss-poor job of it. So, any addiction to alcohol that I developed over the years, cannot be blamed on life's difficulties that arose along the way. I was a crazy drinker from day one.

Whether that little flaw is in my genes, part of the DNA of my notoriously drunken heritage, or I'm just prone to biting life off in chunks of great excess, I do not know. It's almost a moot point. All I know is that I consistently drank way over my allotted limit, and did so from the very beginning.

———

"So…this Irishman walks out of a bar…"

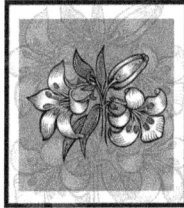

Family, Friends, and Damaged Relationships
HURTING THOSE WE LOVE

I have four children, all grown now, from a previous marriage. I often lament how much emotional damage I inflicted upon them due to my drinking. I never abused them physically, as I know often happens with heavy drinkers, but the emotional and psychological trauma, the sadness and emptiness of a broken family…it takes a severe toll on everyone. Kids especially. I know I caused them a lot of pain and for that I am truly sorry.

Their mother was and still is a very frightened, narrow-minded person. I don't say that out of any animosity, it's just a fact. While my drinking at the time of our marriage was marginal, she would have nothing to do with alcohol or even entertain the idea that perhaps, if there was a problem, she should stand by me in the midst it. I would not hold it against her, except that it was her own fears, inhibitions and identity problems that lead to the dissolution of our marriage, having nothing to do with alcohol.

Regardless, my fault, hers, or both…it was my children who paid the ultimate price, and for that, I can only take responsibility. I did my very best to take care of them, far above and beyond the legal financial requirements placed upon me. Even still, though, they were forced to grow up without a father under their roof. Nothing I could do could fix that.

My current wife, Karin, is a different story altogether. Married now almost twenty years, my drinking did begin to create problems between us. She couldn't rely on me coming home in the evenings, at least not until very late and more and more, completely drunk, stumbling through the front door, angry and pissed off at the world for being so unfair to me. She put up with a lot from me over the years. Again, no physical abuse, but a lot of emotional turmoil and certainly not the husband she thought she had married.

Karin, however, stuck it out. She stood by me, and not in a classic "enabler" sort of way. Far from it. She is a quiet, strong woman and stood her ground. Hers was more of a commitment to our commitment, if you will, in that she had vowed, "for better or worse, in sickness and health…" and despite her feelings, that's exactly what she was going to do. Fortunately, for us both, we went through the fire together, and came out the other side, still together. I love her for that and truly sorry for the pain I caused her in life.

I tried as best I could to hide my problem drinking from others. As a result, other than causing a raised eyebrow now and then, along with no uncertain amount of worry and concern, my addiction had little negative affect on the lives of my friends and business associates. Many problem-drinkers cannot tell the same story and drinking often destroys all their relationships one after the other. Somehow, I escaped that.

I often remember a man who lived across the street from my when I was a small boy. My mother told me, "Poor Wally…he's an alcoholic." I didn't know what this meant, but knew he was not the sort of man that was safe. He scared the daylights out of me, as though I might become infected with whatever strange disease he had. (Maybe I did.)

One day, my mother was visiting with his wife in their living room. Looking back now, I can clearly see he was smashed when he noticed, like any healthy boy, I had dirt under my fingernails. He lifted me up, sat me on his lap and proceeded to remove a pocket knife from his pocket, opening the blade and kindly scraping the dirt from beneath my nails.

I was terrified. I couldn't breathe, let alone call for my mother. I was certain he was going to murder me with that little knife. Isn't that, after all, what alcoholics do? Kill little boys with pocket knives? I was sure of it. Somehow, by the grace of God, I escaped with my life, and some very clean fingernails, I might add.

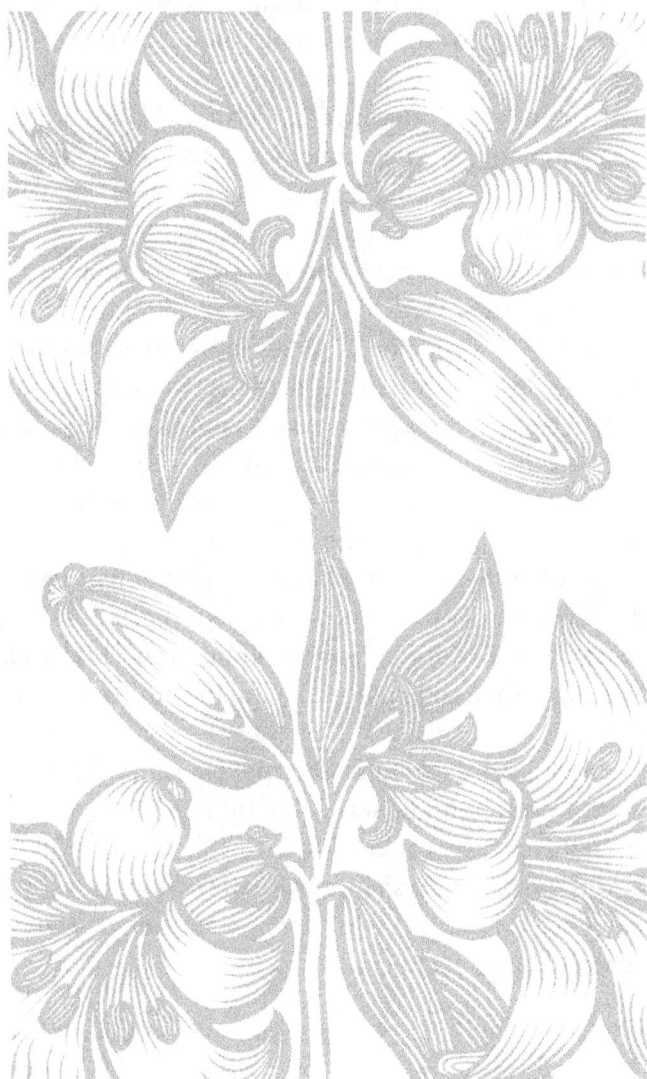

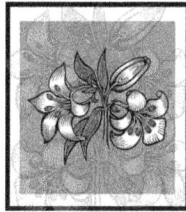

Putting the Puzzle Pieces Together
NOW WHAT DO I DO?

When attending my court-mandated "Drunky Classes," or the esteemed drunk-driving school, I assumed they would have some sort of curriculum or organized program designed to help people. I was so wrong.

The only thing that remotely resembled organization was a retarded form of organized crime. They were very efficient about collecting my money. But anything else was a complete fiasco. Not only was the program not organized around reaching people who may have alcohol problems, but those who were still working on getting there, those individuals who might still have a chance to steer in another direction, they never came close to opening their eyes.

In addition to my hot summer days exploring the old graveyard, this book was also born from that experience. I was looking for answers and the very place that was supposed to provide them, simply didn't care. They had an ongoing, consistent stream of legally-bound, court-mandated, captive audience of paying customers...there was no need to provide a quality service in return. It was sad to witness. It was sadder still, to have to sit through it for over a year and endure the pain.

If my expectation, however, was that the program was simply there to cause more pain and irritation, then I suppose it did its job. Combined with my entire experience, it provided a larger sense of clarity that I was not the only one in the world having to endure all these things and how so many people, good people, well-meaning, hard-working people, have a problem with alcohol. As a society, we know it's far beyond an epidemic. But we laugh it off. The very people who can do something to help, the law-makers, the senators, the judges, the people in high places who get to tell everyone else what to do...they are all likely alcoholics themselves. There are so many people walking around asleep, blind to the sneaky ways in which alcohol robs us all of being alive.

As for me, I don't know anything. Not really. I've only been awake now for a little under three years. That's a great accomplishment in my life, but not enough that I can pretend I'm clear of danger and the ever-sexy lure of a good martini. I'm not stupid. If I've learned one thing along the way, it's how to step back and be aware, listening and identifying that often quiet voice, pretending to be my best friend, concerned with my right to drink when I'm stressed, reminding me how much fun it was. That voice is always there, smaller and more in the background than it used to be, but I know it's still there, keeping a low profile for now, waiting for the right opportunity to pull me aside and talk some sense into me.

But I know that voice is merely the voice of my addiction. It doesn't care about me. It doesn't care about anybody. All it wants is to get drunk. The other stuff, the pain of ruined lives, the financial disaster, the derailed train called my life, they are irrelevant. Grabbing a cocktail and getting smashed is the one and only priority. It's not evil. It's not good or bad. It's simply just addiction, my pre-wired, re-wired, computer-programmed set of brain patterns that do a damn good job of providing me constant direction whether it's helpful or not, whether I want it or not. The only difference now is that I'm aware of it and trying to choose a different route, re-programming myself along the way.

So, what about you?

Does alcohol have a place in your life that has continued to damage your potential as the person you know you could be? Has it strained or ruined relationships? Has it made you late for work more than once? Or landed you in jail? I think, if you're completely honest with yourself and ask whether or not it is time to quit drinking, then in total silence, listen to that voice in your head and see how it responds. Is it nervous? Does it become agitated and self-righteous, declaring your right to drink, swearing you of all people don't have a problem. Yes, maybe others, but not you. Or perhaps it laughs and readily admits there is a problem but then quickly assures you there is also no way in hell you could ever quit drinking. Listen to that voice. Is it really a friend with good advice, or just an addiction struggling to hold on to its only source for a drink?

I think if we really listen to that voice and are brutally honest with ourselves, it isn't that difficult. We know when we have a problem. We may not admit it to others just yet, but if we want the most out of life, we have to admit it to ourselves first.

Life is so short. I for one, don't want to spend it in a dark bar room. Not anymore. I sure as hell don't want to spend it in jail. The high cost of an addiction to alcohol is not worth it, not to me. The return on investment, so to speak, is laughable. But we know that, and we have for quite some time, and yet, we drink anyway.

I don't want to preach to you or anyone. I'm not someone with all the answers. I just know what I'm going through and can see pretty clearly for the first time how I got here. I can hear that old voice now for what it is and, in that clarity, have gained a little more strength to identify it and tell it to shut the hell up. I've seen the damage alcohol can do in people's lives and I've seen what it has done in mine. I don't know why, a smart man like me, would ever allow such a stupid thing to control me, yet I did. For lack of clarity, out of fear, and for the need to eliminate any sign of pain…it promised a solution. And I believed it.

Not anymore. I can't. My hope and my prayer are that my eyes will stay open. That I won't fall back asleep and forget what I have seen. My desire would be that you, too, could realize the same. That maybe, in some small way, my struggles, leading me through the fire, gaining little nuggets of insight, might help you as well. Even just a little.

Please…rise up from that grave you have been lying in for so long. You're not dead yet. You don't belong there. Wake up. The sun is out and it's a beautiful day. There's so much to do still. You've been asleep for so long now.

It's time to wake up.

———————————

SPECIAL THANKS

I'd like to offer a deep debt of gratitude to my friend and therapist, Dr. Kurt Smith. He listened to me banter on for hours about how the world is so unfair to me, but always helped steer me down a better road. As a counselor, he has a real gift for listening to what is really being said and revealing how that often holds me back.

I'd also like to thank my wife, Karin, for her enduring love and support. I put her through Hell and for some reason she stayed by me.

My business partner, Matt Kolbert, also stood by me, believing in me, and in everything he says and does, is committed to my personal success and happiness in life, seemingly more than his own. He is a true friend.

I have many other dear friends who also stood by my side throughout my ordeal, Chris, Ian, Garth and others. My sister Terry and brother John, for always being there, always solid rocks, always my closest allies…thank you.

But most of all, I want to thank my children, Ethan, Marissa, Elle, and Forrest, apologize for the needless pain you have endured by my mistakes, and commit myself to loving you and being available to you in life. Have lots of grandbabies for me. I promise you will never have to worry about having them around a drunken Grandpa.

Finally, my two younger boys, Gerrit and Hardy. You two goofballs will not have to grow up in a world of needless hurt and confusion brought on by a drinking father. You will get my very best, and for that, I am truly a happy man.

God bless you all.

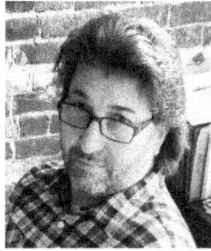

About the Author

David Flanagan is a rather strange entrepreneurial mixture of businessman, writer, speaker and artist. Having grown several successful advertising agencies, since the early 1980's he has established a reputation for cutting against the grain in just about everything to which he lays his hand.

In addition, he spent several years pursuing his passions in the world of filmmaking, developing and producing a handful of independent feature films with box office stars such as Charlize Theron, Michelle Rodriguez, Vivica Fox, Matthew Perry, Rumer Willis, Rob Schneider and more.

Today, as the father of six children, he spends his time writing, speaking across the country, and growing an award-winning brand and marketing agency appropriately named… *Misfit*.

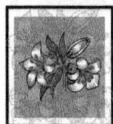

David can be reached at dflanaganbz@gmail.com
Speaking engagements can also be secured by visiting
FlanaganSpeaks.com